Welcome to *"5-Ingredient Diverticulitis-Friendly Meals: 110+ Simple Recipes"*. This book is your essential guide to managing diverticulitis with ease, flavor, and minimal effort. Whether you are newly diagnosed or have been living with diverticulitis for years, finding meals that are both delicious and gentle on your digestive system can be a challenge. This cookbook is designed to simplify that process.

Why 5 Ingredients?

I0477642

We understand that life can be hectic, and cooking elaborate meals is not always feasible. That's why all the recipes in this book are crafted with just five ingredients or fewer. This approach not only saves you time and reduces stress in the kitchen but also ensures that your meals are straightforward and nourishing.

Focus on Diverticulitis-Friendly Foods

Each recipe in this collection has been carefully developed to meet the dietary needs of those with diverticulitis. We emphasize ingredients that are easy to digest, high in fiber (where appropriate), and low in fat. Our goal is to help you manage your symptoms, prevent flare-ups, and enjoy food again.

Simple, Delicious, and Nutritious

Healthy eating doesn't have to be bland or boring. Our recipes are packed with flavor and nutrition, proving that you can enjoy delicious meals while taking care of your digestive health. From hearty breakfasts and satisfying lunches to comforting dinners and delightful desserts, you'll find a variety of options to suit every taste and occasion.

What to Expect
In this book, you'll find:
- Breakfast Recipes: Start your day with easy, energizing meals.
- Lunch and Dinner Recipes: Discover a range of main courses that are quick to prepare and full of flavor.
- Snacks and Sides: Enjoy simple, healthy bites between meals.
- Desserts: Indulge in sweet treats that won't disrupt your diet.

Each recipe includes clear instructions, nutritional information, and tips for ingredient substitutions, ensuring you have everything you need to create meals that are both enjoyable and diverticulitis-friendly.

Thank you for choosing "5-Ingredient Diverticulitis-Friendly Meals: 110+ Simple Recipes." Here's to happy, healthy cooking!

1. Scrambled Eggs: Eggs, milk, butter, salt, pepper.

Ingredients:

• 4 eggs
• 2 tablespoons milk
• 1 teaspoon butter
• 1/4 teaspoon salt
• 1/8 teaspoon ground black pepper

Instructions:

1. Crack the eggs into a small bowl and whisk them together with the milk until well combined.

2. Melt the butter in a nonstick skillet over medium heat.

3. Pour the egg mixture into the skillet and let it sit for 20•30 seconds to set the bottom slightly.

4. Using a spatula, gently push the eggs from the side of the pan into the center, tilting the pan to allow the uncooked egg to flow to the edges.

5. Continue this process, gently folding and stirring the eggs, until they are softly scrambled and cooked through, about 2•3 minutes total.

6. Remove from heat and season with salt and pepper.

7. Serve immediately.

The key things that make this recipe diverticulitis•friendly are:
• Using a small amount of milk instead of cream or cheese
• Avoiding any high•fiber ingredients like vegetables
• Keeping the seasoning simple with just salt and pepper

This simple scrambled egg dish is easy to digest and gentle on the digestive system.

2. Greek Yogurt with Honey: Greek yogurt, honey.

Ingredients:

• 1 cup plain Greek yogurt
• 2 tablespoons honey

Instructions:

1. Scoop the Greek yogurt into a bowl.

2. Drizzle the honey over the top of the yogurt.

3. Gently stir the honey into the yogurt until well combined.

That's it! This easy, 2•ingredient dish is a great option for those with diverticulitis for a few reasons:

1. Greek yogurt is low in fiber and easy to digest, unlike regular yogurt.

2. Honey is a simple, natural sweetener that is gentle on the digestive system.

3. There are no other ingredients that could potentially aggravate diverticulitis, like nuts, seeds, or high•fiber fruits/vegetables.

The combination of protein•rich Greek yogurt and soothing honey makes this a nutritious and easily digestible snack or light meal for those managing diverticulitis. The small number of ingredients also makes it a quick and convenient option.

3. Oatmeal with Banana:
Oats, water, banana, honey, cinnamon.

Ingredients:

• 1/2 cup rolled oats
• 1 cup water
• 1 ripe banana, mashed
• 1 tablespoon honey
• 1/4 teaspoon ground cinnamon

Instructions:

1. In a small saucepan, combine the rolled oats and water. Bring to a boil over medium heat.

2. Reduce heat to low and simmer, stirring occasionally, until the oats are tender and have reached your desired consistency, about 5•7 minutes.

3. Remove the oatmeal from heat and stir in the mashed banana, honey, and cinnamon until well combined. Serve warm.

This oatmeal recipe is diverticulitis•friendly for a few reasons:

1. Rolled oats are a low•fiber, easy•to•digest whole grain.

2. Bananas are a soft, low•fiber fruit that won't aggravate diverticulitis.

3. Honey is a gentle, natural sweetener.

4. Cinnamon adds flavor without any fiber.

5. The recipe uses a small number of simple, whole food ingredients.

The combination of creamy oats, sweet banana, and warming spices makes this a comforting and nourishing breakfast or snack for those managing diverticulitis. The small number of ingredients also makes it easy to prepare.

4. Smoothie:
Banana, almond milk, blueberries, honey.

Ingredients:

• 1 ripe banana, frozen
• 1 cup unsweetened almond milk
• 1/2 cup fresh or frozen blueberries
• 1 tablespoon honey

Instructions:

1. Add the frozen banana, almond milk, blueberries, and honey to a high•powered blender.

2. Blend on high speed until smooth and creamy, about 1•2 minutes.

3. Pour into a glass and enjoy immediately.

This smoothie is diverticulitis•friendly for the following reasons:

1. Bananas are a low•fiber, easy•to•digest fruit.

2. Almond milk is gentle on the digestive system, unlike dairy milk.

3. Blueberries are a low•fiber berry that can be well•tolerated.

4. Honey is a simple, natural sweetener.

5. The recipe uses only 4 whole food ingredients, keeping it simple and easy to digest.

The combination of creamy banana, sweet blueberries, and soothing almond milk makes this a nourishing and satisfying smoothie for those managing diverticulitis. The small number of ingredients also makes it quick and easy to prepare.

5. Poached Eggs on White Toast: Eggs, white bread, butter, salt.

Ingredients:

1. Eggs
2. White bread (soft, crustless)
3. Butter (or a dairy•free alternative)
4. Salt

Instructions:

1. Bring a pot of water to a gentle simmer. Crack the eggs one at a time into the simmering water and poach for 3•5 minutes, until the whites are set but the yolks are still runny.

2. Toast the white bread and spread a small amount of butter on each slice.

3. Carefully remove the poached eggs from the water using a slotted spoon and place them on the buttered toast.

4. Season with a pinch of salt.

Tips for Diverticulitis:

• White bread is easier to digest than whole grain bread for those with diverticulitis.

• Butter is well•tolerated, but you can use a dairy•free alternative if preferred.

• Poached eggs are gentle on the digestive system compared to fried or scrambled eggs.

• Avoid any additional toppings or seasonings that could be irritating, such as pepper or herbs.

This simple, 5•ingredient meal provides protein from the eggs and is easy on the digestive system, making it a suitable option for those managing diverticulitis.

6. Apple Sauce: Apples, sugar, water, cinnamon.

Ingredients:

1. Apples, peeled, cored, and chopped (about 4•5 medium apples)
2. Water
3. Granulated sugar (or honey)
4. Ground cinnamon
5. Lemon juice (optional)

Instructions:

1. In a medium saucepan, combine the chopped apples and just enough water to cover the bottom of the pan, about 1/4 cup.

2. Bring the mixture to a simmer over medium heat, then reduce the heat to low, cover, and cook for 15•20 minutes, stirring occasionally, until the apples are very soft.

3. Remove the lid and continue cooking for 5•10 minutes, stirring frequently, until the apples have broken down into a chunky applesauce consistency.

4. Remove the pan from the heat and stir in the sugar (or honey) and ground cinnamon to taste. Start with 2•3 tablespoons of sugar and 1/2 teaspoon of cinnamon, then adjust to your preference.

5. For a smoother texture, you can use a potato masher or immersion blender to puree the applesauce further.

6. If desired, stir in a teaspoon or two of lemon juice to help balance the sweetness.

Tips for Diverticulitis:

• Peeled, cooked apples are easy to digest and gentle on the digestive system.

• Avoid any additional spices or ingredients that could be irritating, such as nutmeg or cloves.

• The simple combination of apples, sugar, and cinnamon is soothing and well•tolerated.

• Serve the applesauce warm or chilled, as a side dish or snack.

This 5•ingredient applesauce recipe is a great option for those managing diverticulitis.

7. Rice Pudding:
White rice, milk, sugar, vanilla extract.

Ingredients:

1. White rice (short•grain or arborio)
2. Milk (dairy or non•dairy)
3. Granulated sugar
4. Vanilla extract
5. Cinnamon (optional)

Instructions:

1. In a medium saucepan, combine the rice and milk. Bring the mixture to a gentle simmer over medium heat, stirring occasionally.

2. Reduce the heat to low and continue cooking, stirring frequently, for 20•25 minutes, or until the rice is tender and the mixture has thickened to a creamy consistency.

3. Stir in the sugar and vanilla extract, adjusting the amounts to your taste preference.

4. If desired, sprinkle a small amount of ground cinnamon on top of the rice pudding. Serve the rice pudding warm or chilled.

Tips for Diverticulitis:

• White rice is easier to digest than brown rice for those with diverticulitis.

• Milk provides a creamy texture and additional nutrients, but you can use a non•dairy milk alternative if preferred.

• Sugar and vanilla extract add sweetness and flavor without any potentially irritating spices or ingredients.

• Cinnamon is optional, as it may be better to avoid it if you find it to be irritating.

• This simple, 5•ingredient rice pudding is gentle on the digestive system and provides a comforting, nourishing meal or snack.

Remember to adjust the cooking time and consistency of the rice pudding to your personal preference. Enjoy this diverticulitis•friendly dessert or breakfast option.

8. Boiled Eggs: Eggs, salt.

Ingredients:

1. Eggs
2. Salt (optional)

Instructions:

1. Place the eggs in a single layer in a saucepan and cover with cold water by about 1 inch.

2. Bring the water to a boil over high heat.

3. Once the water reaches a rolling boil, remove the pan from the heat and cover with a lid.

4. Let the eggs sit in the hot water for the desired doneness:
   • For soft•boiled eggs: 3•5 minutes
   • For hard•boiled eggs: 10•12 minutes

5. Drain the hot water and cover the eggs with cold water to stop the cooking process.

6. Peel the eggs and season with a pinch of salt, if desired.

Tips for Diverticulitis:

• Boiled eggs are easy to digest and gentle on the digestive system.

• Avoid any additional seasonings or toppings that could be irritating, such as pepper or herbs.

• Salt is optional, as some people with diverticulitis may need to limit their sodium intake.

• Serve the boiled eggs as a simple, protein•rich snack or part of a larger diverticulitis•friendly meal.

This 2•ingredient boiled egg recipe is a great option for those managing diverticulitis, providing a nutritious and easily digestible food.

9. Mashed Avocado on Toast:
Avocado, white bread, lemon juice, salt.

Ingredients:

1. Avocado
2. White bread (soft, crustless)
3. Lemon juice
4. Salt
5. Olive oil (optional)

Instructions:

1. Mash the avocado in a bowl with a fork until it reaches your desired consistency.

2. Add a squeeze of lemon juice and a pinch of salt, and mix well.

3. Toast the white bread until lightly golden.

4. Spread the mashed avocado evenly over the toasted bread slices.

5. If desired, drizzle a small amount of olive oil over the avocado toast.

Tips for Diverticulitis:

• Avocado is a gentle, fiber•rich food that is well•tolerated by those with diverticulitis.

• White bread is easier to digest than whole grain bread for those with diverticulitis.

• Lemon juice helps to balance the richness of the avocado and provides a touch of acidity.

• Salt is used sparingly to enhance the flavors without being overpowering.

• Olive oil is optional, as some people with diverticulitis may prefer to avoid it.

• Avoid any additional toppings or seasonings that could be irritating, such as pepper or herbs.

This 5•ingredient mashed avocado on toast is a simple, nutritious, and diverticulitis•friendly meal or snack option.

10. Cream of Wheat:
Cream of wheat, milk, sugar, butter.

Ingredients:

1. Cream of Wheat (or other farina cereal)
2. Milk (dairy or non•dairy)
3. Granulated sugar
4. Butter (or dairy•free alternative)
5. Salt (optional)

Instructions:

1. In a medium saucepan, bring the milk to a gentle simmer over medium heat.

2. Slowly whisk in the Cream of Wheat, stirring constantly to prevent lumps from forming.

3. Reduce the heat to low and continue cooking, stirring frequently, for 5•7 minutes, or until the Cream of Wheat has thickened to your desired consistency.

4. Remove the pan from the heat and stir in the sugar and a pinch of salt (if using).

5. Serve the Cream of Wheat warm, with a small pat of butter on top.

Tips for Diverticulitis:

• Cream of Wheat is a smooth, easy•to•digest cereal that is gentle on the digestive system.

• Milk provides creaminess and additional nutrients, but you can use a non•dairy milk alternative if preferred.

• Sugar adds a touch of sweetness, but you can adjust the amount to your taste preference.

• Butter (or a dairy•free alternative) adds richness and flavor, but it can be omitted if desired.

• Salt is optional, as some people with diverticulitis may need to limit their sodium intake.

• Avoid any additional toppings or mix•ins that could be irritating, such as nuts, dried fruit, or spices.

This 5•ingredient Cream of Wheat recipe is a comforting, nourishing, and diverticulitis•friendly breakfast or snack option.

11. Chicken and Rice Soup: Chicken breast, white rice, carrots, celery, broth.

Ingredients:

1. Boneless, skinless chicken breasts
2. White rice
3. Carrots, peeled and sliced
4. Celery, sliced
5. Chicken broth

Instructions:

1. In a large pot or Dutch oven, bring the chicken broth to a simmer over medium heat.

2. Add the chicken breasts and simmer for 15•20 minutes, or until the chicken is cooked through.

3. Remove the chicken from the broth and shred or chop it into bite•sized pieces.

4. Return the shredded chicken to the pot and add the sliced carrots and celery.

5. Stir in the white rice and continue simmering for 15•20 minutes, or until the rice and vegetables are tender.

6. Season with salt and pepper to taste, if desired.

Tips for Diverticulitis:

• Chicken breast is a lean protein that is easy to digest.

• White rice is more gentle on the digestive system than brown rice.

• Carrots and celery provide nutrients without being overly fibrous.

• Chicken broth is a soothing, hydrating base for the soup.

• Avoid any additional herbs, spices, or ingredients that could be irritating, such as onions or garlic.

This 5•ingredient Chicken and Rice Soup is a comforting, nourishing, and diverticulitis•friendly meal. Adjust the cooking time and seasoning to your personal preferences.

12. Tuna Salad: Canned tuna, mayonnaise, salt, pepper, lemon juice.

Ingredients:

1. Canned tuna, drained
2. Mayonnaise (or a dairy•free alternative)
3. Lemon juice
4. Salt
5. Ground black pepper (optional)

Instructions:

1. In a medium bowl, flake the drained tuna with a fork.

2. Add the mayonnaise and lemon juice, and mix well until the tuna is evenly coated.

3. Season with a pinch of salt and a small amount of ground black pepper, if desired.

4. Stir the tuna salad until all the ingredients are well combined.

Tips for Diverticulitis:

• Canned tuna is a lean protein that is easy to digest.

• Mayonnaise provides creaminess and helps bind the tuna salad together. You can use a dairy•free alternative if preferred.

• Lemon juice adds a touch of acidity to balance the richness of the mayonnaise.

• Salt is used sparingly to enhance the flavors without being overpowering.

• Ground black pepper is optional, as some people with diverticulitis may find it irritating.

• Avoid any additional ingredients, such as onions, celery, or relish, that could be difficult to digest.

This 5•ingredient tuna salad is a simple, protein•rich option that is gentle on the digestive system for those with diverticulitis. Serve it on a bed of lettuce, on top of crackers, or with a side of white bread.

13. Egg Salad Sandwich:
Eggs, mayonnaise, white bread, salt, pepper.

Ingredients:

1. Hard•boiled eggs, peeled and chopped
2. Mayonnaise (or a dairy•free alternative)
3. White bread, toasted
4. Salt
5. Ground black pepper (optional)

Instructions:

1. In a medium bowl, gently mix the chopped hard•boiled eggs with the mayonnaise until well combined.

2. Season the egg salad with a pinch of salt and a small amount of ground black pepper, if desired.

3. Toast the white bread slices until lightly golden.

4. Spread the egg salad evenly over one slice of toast. Top with the other slice of toast to create a sandwich.

Tips for Diverticulitis:
• Hard•boiled eggs are easy to digest and a gentle protein source.

• Mayonnaise provides creaminess and helps bind the egg salad together. You can use a dairy•free alternative if preferred.

• White bread is more easily tolerated than whole grain bread for those with diverticulitis.

• Salt is used sparingly to enhance the flavors without being overpowering.

• Ground black pepper is optional, as some people with diverticulitis may find it irritating.

• Avoid any additional ingredients, such as onions, celery, or relish, that could be difficult to digest.

This 5•ingredient egg salad sandwich is a simple, nourishing, and diverticulitis•friendly meal or snack option.

14. Turkey Sandwich:
Turkey breast, white bread, mayonnaise, lettuce.

Ingredients:

1. Sliced turkey breast
2. White bread, toasted
3. Mayonnaise (or a dairy•free alternative)
4. Lettuce leaves
5. Salt (optional)

Instructions:

1. Toast the white bread slices until lightly golden.

2. Spread a thin layer of mayonnaise on one slice of toast.

3. Layer the sliced turkey breast on top of the mayonnaise.

4. Place a few lettuce leaves on top of the turkey.

5. Top with the other slice of toast to create the sandwich.

6. If desired, season the sandwich with a pinch of salt.

Tips for Diverticulitis:

• Turkey breast is a lean, easily digestible protein.

• White bread is more gentle on the digestive system than whole grain bread.

• Mayonnaise provides creaminess and helps hold the sandwich together. You can use a dairy•free alternative if preferred.

• Lettuce leaves add a crisp, refreshing texture without being overly fibrous.

• Salt is optional, as some people with diverticulitis may need to limit their sodium intake.

• Avoid any additional ingredients, such as tomatoes, onions, or condiments, that could be irritating.

This 5•ingredient turkey sandwich is a simple, nourishing, and diverticulitis•friendly meal option. Adjust the fillings to your personal preferences and dietary needs.

15. Broth•Based Soup:
Chicken broth, noodles, carrots, celery, salt.

Ingredients:

1. Chicken broth
2. Egg noodles (or other small, soft pasta)
3. Carrots, peeled and sliced
4. Celery, sliced
5. Salt (optional)

Instructions:

1. In a large pot, bring the chicken broth to a gentle simmer over medium heat.

2. Add the egg noodles and continue simmering for 5•7 minutes, or until the noodles are tender.

3. Add the sliced carrots and celery to the pot and continue cooking for an additional 5•10 minutes, or until the vegetables are tender.

4. Season the soup with a pinch of salt, if desired.

5. Serve the broth•based soup warm.

Tips for Diverticulitis:

• Chicken broth provides a soothing, hydrating base for the soup.

• Egg noodles are a soft, easy•to•digest pasta option.

• Carrots and celery add nutrients without being overly fibrous.

• Salt is used sparingly, as some people with diverticulitis may need to limit their sodium intake.

• Avoid any additional ingredients, such as onions, herbs, or spices, that could be irritating.

This 5•ingredient broth•based soup is a simple, nourishing, and diverticulitis•friendly meal. Adjust the cooking time and seasoning to your personal preferences.

16. Baked Chicken Breast: Chicken breast, olive oil, salt, pepper, lemon.

Ingredients:

1. Boneless, skinless chicken breasts
2. Olive oil (or a neutral oil)
3. Salt
4. Ground black pepper (optional)
5. Lemon wedges (for serving)

Instructions:

1. Preheat your oven to 400°F (200°C).

2. Pat the chicken breasts dry with paper towels and place them in a baking dish or on a rimmed baking sheet.

3. Drizzle the chicken with a small amount of olive oil and use your hands or a brush to lightly coat the chicken on all sides.

4. Season the chicken with a pinch of salt and a small amount of ground black pepper, if desired.

5. Bake the chicken for 20•25 minutes, or until it reaches an internal temperature of 165°F (75°C). Serve the baked chicken breast warm, with lemon wedges on the side.

Tips for Diverticulitis:
• Chicken breast is a lean, easily digestible protein.

• Olive oil provides a small amount of healthy fat without being overly rich.

• Salt is used sparingly to enhance the flavors without being overpowering.

• Ground black pepper is optional, as some people with diverticulitis may find it irritating.

• Lemon wedges add a refreshing, acidic note that can help balance the dish.

• Avoid any additional seasonings, herbs, or sauces that could be difficult to digest.

This 5•ingredient baked chicken breast recipe is a simple, nourishing, and diverticulitis•friendly main dish. Adjust the cooking time as needed to ensure the chicken is cooked through.

17. Mashed Potatoes:
Potatoes, butter, milk, salt, pepper.

Ingredients:

1. Potatoes, peeled and cut into 1•inch cubes
2. Butter (or a dairy•free alternative)
3. Milk (dairy or non•dairy)
4. Salt
5. Ground black pepper (optional)

Instructions:

1. Place the cubed potatoes in a large pot and cover with cold water.

2. Bring the water to a boil over high heat, then reduce the heat to medium•low and simmer for 15•20 minutes, or until the potatoes are very tender when pierced with a fork.

3. Drain the potatoes and return them to the pot.

4. Add a small amount of butter and a splash of milk, and mash the potatoes with a potato masher or electric mixer until smooth and creamy.

5. Season the mashed potatoes with a pinch of salt and a small amount of ground black pepper, if desired. Serve the mashed potatoes warm.

Tips for Diverticulitis:
• Potatoes are a gentle, starchy vegetable that is easy to digest.

• Butter (or a dairy•free alternative) adds richness and creaminess to the mashed potatoes.

• Milk provides additional moisture and a creamy texture. You can use a non•dairy milk if preferred.

• Salt is used sparingly to enhance the flavors without being overpowering.

• Ground black pepper is optional, as some people with diverticulitis may find it irritating. Avoid any additional ingredients, such as garlic, onions, or herbs, that could be difficult to digest.

This 5•ingredient mashed potato recipe is a comforting, nourishing, and diverticulitis•friendly side dish. Adjust the amounts of butter and milk to achieve your desired consistency.

18. Rice and Chicken Bowl:
White rice, grilled chicken, soy sauce, peas, carrots.

Ingredients:

1. White rice
2. Grilled or baked chicken breasts, sliced or shredded
3. Soy sauce (or a low•sodium alternative)
4. Frozen peas
5. Carrots, peeled and sliced

Instructions:

1. Cook the white rice according to the package instructions.

2. In a large skillet or saucepan, combine the sliced or shredded chicken and a small amount of soy sauce. Heat the chicken through, stirring occasionally.

3. Add the frozen peas and sliced carrots to the skillet with the chicken. Cook for 5•7 minutes, or until the vegetables are tender.

4. Serve the chicken and vegetable mixture over the cooked white rice.

5. Drizzle a small amount of additional soy sauce over the top, if desired.

Tips for Diverticulitis:

• White rice is easier to digest than brown rice for those with diverticulitis.

• Grilled or baked chicken breast is a lean, easily digestible protein.

• Soy sauce adds flavor without being overly spicy or acidic.

• Frozen peas and carrots provide nutrients without being too fibrous.

• Avoid any additional ingredients, such as onions, garlic, or other seasonings, that could be irritating.

This 5•ingredient Rice and Chicken Bowl is a simple, nourishing, and diverticulitis•friendly meal. Adjust the amounts of each ingredient to your personal preferences and dietary needs.

19. Grilled Cheese Sandwich:
White bread, cheese, butter.

Ingredients:

1. White bread
2. Cheese (such as cheddar or American)
3. Butter (or a dairy•free alternative)

Instructions:

1. Lightly butter one side of each slice of bread.

2. Place one slice of bread, butter•side down, in a skillet or griddle over medium heat.

3. Top the bread with slices of cheese, then place the other slice of bread, butter•side up, on top.

4. Cook the sandwich for 2•3 minutes per side, or until the bread is golden brown and the cheese is melted.

5. Carefully flip the sandwich and cook the other side until it's also golden brown.

6. Remove the grilled cheese sandwich from the heat and serve immediately.

Tips for Diverticulitis:

• White bread is easier to digest than whole grain bread for those with diverticulitis.

• Cheese provides a source of protein and calcium without being too heavy or rich.

• Butter (or a dairy•free alternative) helps create a crispy, golden exterior on the bread.

• Avoid any additional ingredients, such as tomatoes, onions, or other toppings, that could be irritating.

This 3•ingredient grilled cheese sandwich is a simple, comforting, and diverticulitis•friendly meal. Adjust the type and amount of cheese to your personal preferences.

20. Salmon and Rice: Salmon fillet, white rice, olive oil, lemon, salt.

Ingredients:

1. Salmon fillet
2. White rice
3. Olive oil
4. Lemon
5. Salt

Instructions:

1. Preheat your oven to 400°F (200°C).

2. Place the salmon fillet on a baking sheet or in a baking dish. Drizzle with a small amount of olive oil and season with a pinch of salt.

3. Bake the salmon for 12•15 minutes, or until it flakes easily with a fork.

4. While the salmon is baking, cook the white rice according to the package instructions.

5. Once the salmon is cooked, flake it into large chunks using a fork.

6. Serve the salmon over the cooked white rice, and squeeze a fresh lemon wedge over the top.

Tips for Diverticulitis:

• Salmon is a lean, omega•3 rich fish that is easy to digest.

• White rice is more gentle on the digestive system than brown rice.

• Olive oil provides a small amount of healthy fat without being overly rich.

• Lemon adds a refreshing, acidic note that can help balance the dish.

• Salt is used sparingly to enhance the flavors without being overpowering.

• Avoid any additional seasonings, herbs, or sauces that could be irritating.

This 5•ingredient Salmon and Rice dish is a simple, nourishing, and diverticulitis•friendly meal. Adjust the cooking time for the salmon as needed to ensure it's cooked through.

21. Baked Cod:
Cod fillet, olive oil, lemon, salt, pepper.

Ingredients:

1. Cod fillet
2. Olive oil
3. Lemon
4. Salt
5. Ground black pepper (optional)

Instructions:

1. Preheat your oven to 400°F (200°C).

2. Place the cod fillet in a baking dish or on a rimmed baking sheet.

3. Drizzle the cod with a small amount of olive oil and use your hands or a brush to lightly coat the fish.

4. Squeeze fresh lemon juice over the top of the cod.

5. Season the cod with a pinch of salt and a small amount of ground black pepper, if desired.

6. Bake the cod for 12•15 minutes, or until it flakes easily with a fork. Serve the baked cod warm, with additional lemon wedges on the side.

Tips for Diverticulitis:

• Cod is a lean, mild•flavored fish that is easy to digest.

• Olive oil provides a small amount of healthy fat without being overly rich.

• Lemon adds a refreshing, acidic note that can help balance the dish.

• Salt is used sparingly to enhance the flavors without being overpowering.

• Ground black pepper is optional, as some people with diverticulitis may find it irritating.

• Avoid any additional seasonings, herbs, or sauces that could be difficult to digest.

This 5•ingredient baked cod recipe is a simple, nourishing, and diverticulitis•friendly main dish. Adjust the cooking time as needed to ensure the cod is cooked through.

22. Chicken Alfredo Pasta: Chicken breast, pasta, Alfredo sauce, parmesan cheese, butter.

Ingredients:

1. Boneless, skinless chicken breasts
2. White pasta (such as fettuccine or linguine)
3. Alfredo sauce (dairy•free or low•fat version)
4. Parmesan cheese (optional)
5. Butter (or a dairy•free alternative)

Instructions:

1. Preheat your oven to 400°F (200°C).

2. Season the chicken breasts with a pinch of salt and pepper, if desired.

3. Bake the chicken for 20•25 minutes, or until it reaches an internal temperature of 165°F (75°C). Shred or slice the cooked chicken.

4. Cook the white pasta according to the package instructions.

5. In a saucepan, warm the Alfredo sauce over low heat, stirring occasionally.

6. Drain the cooked pasta and return it to the pot. Add the shredded chicken and the warm Alfredo sauce, and toss to combine.

7. Serve the Chicken Alfredo Pasta warm, with a small amount of grated Parmesan cheese on top, if desired.

Tips for Diverticulitis:

• Chicken breast is a lean, easily digestible protein.

• White pasta is gentler on the digestive system than whole wheat pasta.

• Alfredo sauce provides a creamy texture without being too heavy or rich. Look for a dairy•free or low•fat version.

• Parmesan cheese is optional, as some people with diverticulitis may need to limit dairy intake.

• Butter (or a dairy•free alternative) can be used to toss the pasta, but it's not essential.Avoid any additional vegetables, herbs, or spices that could be irritating.

23. Steamed Salmon:
Salmon fillet, lemon, dill, salt, pepper.

Ingredients:

1. Salmon fillet
2. Lemon
3. Fresh dill (optional)
4. Salt
5. Ground black pepper (optional)

Instructions:

1. Fill a large pot with about 1 inch of water and bring it to a gentle simmer over medium heat.

2. Place the salmon fillet in a steamer basket or on a heatproof plate that can fit inside the pot without touching the water.

3. Season the salmon with a pinch of salt and a small amount of ground black pepper, if desired.

4. Squeeze fresh lemon juice over the top of the salmon.

5. If using, sprinkle a small amount of fresh dill over the salmon.

6. Place the steamer basket or plate with the salmon into the pot, making sure the water doesn't touch the fish.

7. Cover the pot with a lid and steam the salmon for 10•15 minutes, or until it flakes easily with a fork. Serve the steamed salmon warm, with additional lemon wedges on the side.

Tips for Diverticulitis:
• Salmon is a lean, omega•3 rich fish that is easy to digest.
• Lemon adds a refreshing, acidic note that can help balance the dish.
• Fresh dill is optional, as some people with diverticulitis may find it irritating.
• Salt is used sparingly to enhance the flavors without being overpowering.
• Ground black pepper is optional, as some people with diverticulitis may find it irritating.
• Avoid any additional seasonings, herbs, or sauces that could be difficult to digest.

This 5•ingredient steamed salmon recipe is a simple, nourishing, and diverticulitis•friendly main dish. Adjust the cooking time as needed to ensure the salmon is cooked through.

24. Turkey Meatloaf:
Ground turkey, breadcrumbs, egg, salt, pepper.

Ingredients:

1. Ground turkey
2. Breadcrumbs (or crushed crackers)
3. Egg
4. Salt
5. Ground black pepper (optional)

Instructions:

1. Preheat your oven to 375°F (190°C).

2. In a large bowl, combine the ground turkey, breadcrumbs, and egg. Mix the ingredients together until well incorporated.

3. Season the turkey mixture with a pinch of salt and a small amount of ground black pepper, if desired.

4. Shape the mixture into a loaf and place it in a baking dish or on a rimmed baking sheet.

5. Bake the turkey meatloaf for 45•55 minutes, or until it reaches an internal temperature of 165°F (75°C). Let the meatloaf rest for 5•10 minutes before slicing and serving.

Tips for Diverticulitis:

• Ground turkey is a lean, easily digestible protein.

• Breadcrumbs (or crushed crackers) help bind the meatloaf together without being too dense or heavy.

• Egg acts as a binder and helps hold the meatloaf together.

• Salt is used sparingly to enhance the flavors without being overpowering.

• Ground black pepper is optional, as some people with diverticulitis may find it irritating.

• Avoid any additional ingredients, such as onions, garlic, or herbs, that could be difficult to digest.

This 5•ingredient turkey meatloaf is a simple, nourishing, and diverticulitis•friendly main dish. Serve it with a side of steamed vegetables or a simple salad.

25. Spaghetti and Meatballs: Spaghetti, ground beef, breadcrumbs, egg, marinara sauce.

Ingredients:

1. Spaghetti (white or gluten•free)
2. Ground beef
3. Breadcrumbs (or crushed crackers)
4. Egg
5. Marinara sauce (low•fiber, low•acid version)

Instructions:

1. Cook the spaghetti according to the package instructions.

2. In a bowl, combine the ground beef, breadcrumbs, and egg. Mix the ingredients together until well incorporated.

3. Form the beef mixture into small meatballs, about 1•2 inches in size.

4. In a large skillet or saucepan, heat a small amount of olive oil over medium heat.

5. Add the meatballs to the skillet and cook, turning occasionally, until they are browned on all sides and cooked through, about 10•12 minutes.

6. Drain the cooked spaghetti and transfer it to a serving dish. Pour the marinara sauce over the spaghetti and top with the cooked meatballs.

Tips for Diverticulitis:

• White or gluten•free spaghetti is easier to digest than whole wheat pasta.

• Ground beef is a lean protein that is gentle on the digestive system.

• Breadcrumbs (or crushed crackers) help bind the meatballs without being too dense.

• Egg acts as a binder and helps hold the meatballs together.

• Marinara sauce should be a low•fiber, low•acid version to avoid irritation.

• Avoid any additional vegetables, herbs, or spices that could be difficult to digest.

This 5•ingredient Spaghetti and Meatballs dish is a simplified, diverticulitis•friendly version of the classic meal. Adjust the amounts of each ingredient to your personal preferences.

26. Baked Tilapia:
Tilapia fillet, olive oil, lemon, garlic, salt.

Ingredients:

1. Tilapia fillets
2. Olive oil
3. Lemon
4. Garlic powder (optional)
5. Salt

Instructions:

1. Preheat your oven to 400°F (200°C).

2. Place the tilapia fillets in a baking dish or on a rimmed baking sheet.

3. Drizzle the tilapia with a small amount of olive oil and use your hands or a brush to lightly coat the fish.

4. Squeeze fresh lemon juice over the top of the tilapia.

5. Sprinkle a pinch of salt and a small amount of garlic powder (if using) over the fish.

6. Bake the tilapia for 12•15 minutes, or until it flakes easily with a fork. Serve the baked tilapia warm, with additional lemon wedges on the side.

Tips for Diverticulitis:

• Tilapia is a mild, white fish that is easy to digest.

• Olive oil provides a small amount of healthy fat without being overly rich.

• Lemon adds a refreshing, acidic note that can help balance the dish.

• Garlic powder is optional, as some people with diverticulitis may find it irritating.

• Salt is used sparingly to enhance the flavors without being overpowering.

• Avoid any additional seasonings, herbs, or sauces that could be difficult to digest.

This 5•ingredient baked tilapia recipe is a simple, nourishing, and diverticulitis•friendly main dish. Adjust the cooking time as needed to ensure the fish is cooked through.

27. Rice Pilaf: White rice, chicken broth, butter, onion, garlic.

Ingredients:

1. White rice
2. Chicken broth
3. Butter (or a dairy•free alternative)
4. Onion powder
5. Garlic powder

Instructions:

1. In a medium saucepan, combine the white rice and chicken broth.

2. Bring the mixture to a boil over high heat, then reduce the heat to low, cover, and simmer for 15•20 minutes, or until the rice is tender and the liquid is absorbed.

3. Remove the saucepan from the heat and stir in a small amount of butter (or a dairy•free alternative).

4. Season the rice pilaf with a pinch of onion powder and a small amount of garlic powder, to taste. Fluff the rice with a fork and serve warm.

Tips for Diverticulitis:

• White rice is easier to digest than brown rice for those with diverticulitis.

• Chicken broth provides flavor without being too heavy or rich.

• Butter (or a dairy•free alternative) adds a touch of creaminess and richness.

• Onion powder and garlic powder provide subtle flavor without being overpowering.

• Avoid any additional ingredients, such as fresh onions or garlic, that could be difficult to digest.

This 5•ingredient rice pilaf is a simple, nourishing, and diverticulitis•friendly side dish. Adjust the seasoning to your personal taste preferences.

28. Grilled Chicken Breast: Chicken breast, olive oil, lemon, salt, pepper.

Ingredients:

1. Boneless, skinless chicken breasts
2. Olive oil
3. Lemon
4. Salt
5. Ground black pepper (optional)

Instructions:

1. Preheat your grill or grill pan to medium•high heat.

2. Lightly brush the chicken breasts with olive oil on both sides.

3. Season the chicken with a pinch of salt and a small amount of ground black pepper, if desired.

4. Grill the chicken for 5•7 minutes per side, or until it reaches an internal temperature of 165°F (75°C).

5. Squeeze fresh lemon juice over the grilled chicken breasts.

6. Serve the grilled chicken warm, with additional lemon wedges on the side.

Tips for Diverticulitis:

• Chicken breast is a lean, easily digestible protein.

• Olive oil provides a small amount of healthy fat without being overly rich.

• Lemon adds a refreshing, acidic note that can help balance the dish.

• Salt is used sparingly to enhance the flavors without being overpowering.

• Ground black pepper is optional, as some people with diverticulitis may find it irritating.

• Avoid any additional seasonings, herbs, or sauces that could be difficult to digest.

This 5•ingredient grilled chicken breast recipe is a simple, nourishing, and diverticulitis•friendly main dish. Adjust the cooking time as needed to ensure the chicken is cooked through.

29. Shepherd's Pie:
Ground beef, potatoes, butter, milk, salt.

Ingredients:

1. Ground beef
2. Potatoes, peeled and cubed
3. Butter (or a dairy•free alternative)
4. Milk (dairy or non•dairy)
5. Salt

Instructions:

1. Preheat your oven to 375°F (190°C).

2. In a skillet, cook the ground beef over medium heat until browned and cooked through. Drain any excess fat.

3. In a separate pot, cover the cubed potatoes with water and bring to a boil. Reduce the heat and simmer for 15•20 minutes, or until the potatoes are tender.

4. Drain the cooked potatoes and mash them with a small amount of butter and milk, adding just enough to achieve a creamy consistency. Season with a pinch of salt.

5. Spread the cooked ground beef in the bottom of a baking dish. Top the beef with the mashed potatoes, spreading them evenly.

6. Bake the Shepherd's Pie for 20•25 minutes, or until the potatoes are lightly browned on top. Serve the Shepherd's Pie warm.

Tips for Diverticulitis:

• Ground beef is a lean protein that is easy to digest.

• Potatoes are a gentle, starchy vegetable that is well•tolerated.

• Butter (or a dairy•free alternative) and milk provide creaminess to the mashed potatoes.

• Salt is used sparingly to enhance the flavors without being overpowering.

• Avoid any additional vegetables, herbs, or spices that could be irritating.

This 5•ingredient Shepherd's Pie is a simplified, diverticulitis•friendly version of the classic dish. Adjust the amounts of each ingredient to your personal preferences.

30. Chicken and Broccoli: Chicken breast, broccoli, olive oil, salt, pepper.

Ingredients:

1. Boneless, skinless chicken breasts
2. Broccoli florets
3. Olive oil
4. Salt
5. Ground black pepper (optional)

Instructions:

1. Preheat your oven to 400°F (200°C).

2. Cut the chicken breasts into bite•sized pieces.

3. In a large bowl, toss the chicken pieces and broccoli florets with a small amount of olive oil, just enough to lightly coat them.

4. Season the chicken and broccoli with a pinch of salt and a small amount of ground black pepper, if desired.

5. Spread the chicken and broccoli mixture in a single layer on a baking sheet.

6. Roast the chicken and broccoli in the preheated oven for 20•25 minutes, or until the chicken is cooked through and the broccoli is tender. Serve the Chicken and Broccoli warm.

Tips for Diverticulitis:

• Chicken breast is a lean, easily digestible protein.

• Broccoli is a nutrient•dense vegetable that is relatively low in fiber, making it gentle on the digestive system.

• Olive oil provides a small amount of healthy fat without being overly rich.

• Salt is used sparingly to enhance the flavors without being overpowering.

• Ground black pepper is optional, as some people with diverticulitis may find it irritating.

• Avoid any additional seasonings, sauces, or ingredients that could be difficult to digest.

This 5•ingredient Chicken and Broccoli dish is a simple, nourishing, and diverticulitis•friendly meal. Adjust the cooking time as needed to ensure the chicken is cooked through and the broccoli is tender.

31. Banana Smoothie:
Banana, almond milk, honey, vanilla extract.

Ingredients:

1. Banana, ripe
2. Unsweetened almond milk
3. Honey (optional)
4. Vanilla extract

Instructions:

1. In a blender, combine the ripe banana, almond milk, a drizzle of honey (if using), and a splash of vanilla extract.

2. Blend the ingredients together until smooth and creamy.

3. Pour the banana smoothie into a glass and serve immediately.

Tips for Diverticulitis:

• Banana is a gentle, easily digestible fruit that is well•tolerated by those with diverticulitis.

• Unsweetened almond milk provides a creamy base without being too heavy or rich.

• Honey is optional, as some people with diverticulitis may need to limit their sugar intake.

• Vanilla extract adds a touch of flavor without any irritating spices or ingredients.

• Avoid any additional ingredients, such as yogurt, ice cream, or other fruits, that could be difficult to digest.

This 4•ingredient banana smoothie is a simple, nourishing, and diverticulitis•friendly snack or breakfast option. Adjust the amounts of each ingredient to your personal taste preferences.

32. Cottage Cheese with Peaches: Cottage cheese, canned peaches.

Ingredients:

1. Cottage cheese
2. Canned peach slices (in water or light syrup)

Instructions:

1. Scoop a portion of cottage cheese into a bowl.

2. Top the cottage cheese with a few slices of canned peaches.

3. Serve chilled or at room temperature.

Tips for Diverticulitis:

• Cottage cheese is a gentle, protein•rich dairy product that is well•tolerated by those with diverticulitis.

• Canned peach slices are a soft, easily digestible fruit that provides a touch of sweetness.

• Avoid any additional toppings or ingredients that could be difficult to digest, such as nuts, granola, or fresh fruit.

• If the canned peaches are in heavy syrup, you can drain them or opt for a light syrup or water•packed version to reduce the sugar content.

This 2•ingredient cottage cheese and peaches dish is a simple, nourishing, and diverticulitis•friendly snack or light meal. Adjust the portion sizes to your personal preferences and dietary needs.

33. Rice Cakes with Avocado:
Rice cakes, avocado, salt.

Ingredients:

1. Rice cakes
2. Avocado
3. Salt (optional)

Instructions:

1. Slice or mash the avocado.

2. Spread the avocado evenly over the rice cakes.

3. Season with a pinch of salt, if desired.

Tips for Diverticulitis:

• Rice cakes are a gentle, low•fiber carbohydrate that is easy to digest.

• Avocado is a nutrient•rich, fiber•containing food that is well•tolerated by those with diverticulitis.

• Salt is optional, as some people with diverticulitis may need to limit their sodium intake.

• Avoid any additional toppings or ingredients that could be difficult to digest, such as tomatoes, onions, or spices.

This 3•ingredient rice cakes with avocado snack is a simple, nourishing, and diverticulitis•friendly option. Adjust the amount of avocado to your personal preference.

34. Applesauce: Apples, sugar, water, cinnamon.

Ingredients:

1. Apples, peeled, cored, and chopped
2. Water
3. Granulated sugar (or honey)
4. Ground cinnamon
5. Lemon juice (optional)

Instructions:

1. In a medium saucepan, combine the chopped apples and just enough water to cover the bottom of the pan, about 1/4 cup.

2. Bring the mixture to a simmer over medium heat, then reduce the heat to low, cover, and cook for 15•20 minutes, stirring occasionally, until the apples are very soft.

3. Remove the lid and continue cooking for 5•10 minutes, stirring frequently, until the apples have broken down into a chunky applesauce consistency.

4. Remove the pan from the heat and stir in the sugar (or honey) and ground cinnamon to taste. Start with 2•3 tablespoons of sugar and 1/2 teaspoon of cinnamon, then adjust to your preference.

5. For a smoother texture, you can use a potato masher or immersion blender to puree the applesauce further.

6. If desired, stir in a teaspoon or two of lemon juice to help balance the sweetness.

Tips for Diverticulitis:
• Peeled, cooked apples are easy to digest and gentle on the digestive system.

• The simple combination of apples, sugar, and cinnamon is soothing and well•tolerated.

• Avoid any additional spices or ingredients that could be irritating, such as nutmeg or cloves.

• Serve the applesauce warm or chilled, as a side dish or snack.

This 5•ingredient applesauce recipe is a great option for those managing diverticulitis.

35. Greek Yogurt with Honey: Greek yogurt, honey.

Ingredients:

1. Greek yogurt (plain, low•fat)
2. Honey
3. Blueberries (fresh or frozen)
4. Walnuts (chopped)
5. Cinnamon (ground)

Instructions:

1. Scoop desired amount of Greek yogurt into a bowl.

2. Drizzle honey over the yogurt.

3. Top with fresh or frozen blueberries.

4. Sprinkle chopped walnuts over the top.

5. Lightly dust with ground cinnamon.

This recipe is gentle on the digestive system and provides a good source of protein, probiotics, antioxidants, and healthy fats. The blueberries and walnuts are soft, easy•to•digest ingredients that are recommended for those with diverticulitis. Enjoy this simple, nutritious snack or light meal.

36. Boiled Eggs: Eggs, salt.

Ingredients:

1. Eggs
2. Water
3. Salt
4. Lemon juice
5. Parsley (fresh, chopped)

Instructions:

1. Place the eggs in a single layer in a saucepan and cover with water by 1 inch.

2. Bring the water to a boil over high heat.

3. Once the water is boiling, remove the pan from the heat, cover, and let the eggs sit for 12 minutes.

4. Drain the hot water and cover the eggs with cold water to stop the cooking.

5. Peel the eggs and season with a pinch of salt, a squeeze of lemon juice, and a sprinkle of fresh chopped parsley.

The boiled eggs provide a good source of protein, while the lemon juice and parsley add flavor without being too harsh on the digestive system. This simple recipe is easy to digest and gentle on the diverticulitis•prone gut.

37. Mashed Potatoes: Potatoes, butter, milk, salt.

Ingredients:

1. Potatoes (peeled and cut into 1•inch cubes)
2. Chicken or vegetable broth
3. Garlic (minced)
4. Greek yogurt
5. Salt and pepper to taste

Instructions:

1. Place the cubed potatoes in a saucepan and cover with the broth. Bring to a boil.

2. Reduce heat and simmer for 15•20 minutes, or until the potatoes are tender when pierced with a fork.

3. Drain the potatoes, reserving a small amount of the cooking liquid.

4. In a large bowl, mash the potatoes with a potato masher or electric mixer. Gradually add in the Greek yogurt, minced garlic, and a splash of the reserved cooking liquid until you reach your desired consistency.

5. Season with salt and pepper to taste.

This recipe uses broth instead of milk and butter to keep the mashed potatoes gentle on the digestive system. The Greek yogurt provides creaminess and probiotics, while the garlic adds flavor without being too harsh. This simple, 5•ingredient mashed potato dish is a great option for those with diverticulitis.

38. Plain Popcorn: Popcorn kernels, salt.

Ingredients:

1. Popcorn kernels
2. Olive oil or avocado oil
3. Salt
4. Garlic powder (optional)
5. Dried herbs (such as rosemary or thyme, optional)

Instructions:

1. In a large pot with a tight•fitting lid, heat 2•3 tablespoons of olive oil or avocado oil over medium•high heat.

2. Once the oil is hot, add the popcorn kernels in a single layer. Cover the pot with the lid.

3. Allow the kernels to pop, shaking the pot occasionally to prevent burning. Once the popping slows to 2•3 seconds between pops, remove the pot from the heat.

4. Transfer the popped popcorn to a large bowl. Season with a light sprinkle of salt, and optionally, a dash of garlic powder and/or dried herbs.

5. Toss the popcorn to evenly distribute the seasonings.

This simple popcorn recipe is gentle on the digestive system, as it avoids any butter or heavy seasonings that could irritate the gut. The plain, lightly salted popcorn is a great snack option for those with diverticulitis. You can also experiment with different dried herbs to add flavor without upsetting the stomach.

39. Soft Cheese and Crackers:
Soft cheese, saltine crackers.

Ingredients:

1. Soft cheese (such as ricotta, cottage cheese, or cream cheese)
2. Whole grain crackers (such as Triscuits or Wasa crackers)
3. Grapes (seedless, halved)
4. Honey (optional)
5. Chives or green onions, chopped (optional)

Instructions:

1. Spread a small amount of the soft cheese onto each cracker.

2. Top the cheese•topped crackers with a few halved grapes.

3. Drizzle a small amount of honey over the grapes, if desired.

4. Sprinkle the chopped chives or green onions over the top, if using.

This simple snack provides a balance of protein, carbohydrates, and healthy fats, all of which are gentle on the digestive system. The soft cheese and crackers are easy to digest, while the grapes add a touch of sweetness without being too harsh. The optional honey and herbs add flavor without irritating the gut.

This 5•ingredient snack is a great option for those with diverticulitis, as it is low in fiber and easy on the stomach. Adjust the portion sizes as needed to meet your individual dietary needs.

40. Rice Pudding:
White rice, milk, sugar, vanilla extract.

Ingredients:

1. White rice (short•grain or arborio)
2. Unsweetened almond milk (or dairy milk)
3. Honey (or maple syrup)
4. Cinnamon
5. Vanilla extract

Instructions:

1. In a medium saucepan, combine the rice and almond milk (or dairy milk).

2. Bring the mixture to a simmer over medium heat, stirring occasionally.

3. Reduce the heat to low and continue simmering, stirring frequently, until the rice is tender and the mixture has thickened, about 20•25 minutes.

4. Remove the saucepan from the heat and stir in the honey (or maple syrup) and vanilla extract.

5. Serve the rice pudding warm, sprinkled with a dash of cinnamon.

This rice pudding recipe is gentle on the digestive system, as it uses simple, easy•to•digest ingredients. The almond milk or dairy milk provides creaminess, while the honey or maple syrup adds sweetness without being too harsh. The cinnamon provides a touch of flavor without irritating the gut.

This 5•ingredient rice pudding is a comforting and nourishing dessert or snack option for those with diverticulitis. Adjust the sweetener and spices to your personal taste preferences.

41. Banana Ice Cream:
Bananas, almond milk, honey.

Ingredients:

1. Ripe bananas, frozen
2. Unsweetened almond milk
3. Honey (or maple syrup)
4. Cinnamon
5. Vanilla extract

Instructions:

1. In a high•powered blender or food processor, blend the frozen banana slices until smooth and creamy, scraping down the sides as needed.

2. Add the almond milk, a drizzle of honey (or maple syrup), a sprinkle of cinnamon, and a splash of vanilla extract. Blend again until well combined.

3. Taste and adjust sweetener or spices as desired.

4. Serve immediately for a soft•serve consistency, or transfer to a freezer•safe container and freeze for 2•3 hours for a firmer ice cream texture.

This banana ice cream is a gentle, diverticulitis•friendly dessert. The frozen bananas provide a creamy base, while the almond milk and honey (or maple syrup) add creaminess and sweetness without being too harsh on the digestive system. The cinnamon provides a subtle flavor boost without irritating the gut.

This 5•ingredient recipe is easy to make and can be enjoyed as a healthy, soothing treat for those with diverticulitis. Adjust the sweetener to your taste preferences.

42. Rice Pudding:
White rice, milk, sugar, vanilla extract.

Ingredients:

1. White rice (short•grain or arborio)
2. Unsweetened almond milk (or dairy milk)
3. Honey (or maple syrup)
4. Cinnamon
5. Vanilla extract

Instructions:

1. In a medium saucepan, combine the rice and almond milk (or dairy milk).

2. Bring the mixture to a simmer over medium heat, stirring occasionally.

3. Reduce the heat to low and continue simmering, stirring frequently, until the rice is tender and the mixture has thickened, about 20•25 minutes.

4. Remove the saucepan from the heat and stir in the honey (or maple syrup) and vanilla extract.

5. Serve the rice pudding warm, sprinkled with a dash of cinnamon.

This rice pudding recipe is gentle on the digestive system, as it uses simple, easy•to•digest ingredients. The almond milk or dairy milk provides creaminess, while the honey or maple syrup adds sweetness without being too harsh. The cinnamon provides a touch of flavor without irritating the gut.

This 5•ingredient rice pudding is a comforting and nourishing dessert or snack option for those with diverticulitis. Adjust the sweetener and spices to your personal taste preferences.

43. Vanilla Pudding:
Milk, sugar, cornstarch, vanilla extract.

Ingredients:

1. Unsweetened almond milk (or dairy milk)
2. Honey (or maple syrup)
3. Cornstarch
4. Vanilla extract
5. Cinnamon (optional)

Instructions:

1. In a medium saucepan, whisk together the almond milk (or dairy milk), honey (or maple syrup), and cornstarch until well combined.

2. Place the saucepan over medium heat and cook, stirring constantly, until the mixture thickens and comes to a gentle boil, about 5•7 minutes.

3. Remove the saucepan from the heat and stir in the vanilla extract.

4. Pour the pudding into individual serving dishes or a larger bowl.

5. Refrigerate the pudding for at least 2 hours, or until completely set. Optionally, sprinkle with a light dusting of cinnamon before serving.

This vanilla pudding recipe is gentle on the digestive system, as it uses simple, easy•to•digest ingredients. The almond milk or dairy milk provides the base, while the honey or maple syrup adds sweetness without being too harsh. The cornstarch helps thicken the pudding without adding too much fiber.

The optional cinnamon provides a subtle flavor boost without irritating the gut. This 5•ingredient vanilla pudding is a soothing and nourishing dessert or snack option for those with diverticulitis.

44. Applesauce Cake:
Applesauce, flour, sugar, eggs, baking powder.

Ingredients:

1. Unsweetened applesauce
2. Gluten•free flour (such as almond or oat flour)
3. Honey (or maple syrup)
4. Eggs
5. Baking powder

Instructions:

1. Preheat your oven to 350°F (175°C). Grease a small baking dish or ramekins.

2. In a medium bowl, whisk together the applesauce, gluten•free flour, honey (or maple syrup), and baking powder until well combined.

3. Crack the eggs into the bowl and mix until the batter is smooth and uniform.

4. Pour the batter into the prepared baking dish or ramekins.

5. Bake for 20•25 minutes, or until a toothpick inserted into the center comes out clean.

6. Allow the cake to cool slightly before serving.

This applesauce cake is a gentle, diverticulitis•friendly dessert. The unsweetened applesauce provides moisture and natural sweetness, while the gluten•free flour and honey (or maple syrup) create a tender, easy•to•digest cake. The eggs help bind the ingredients together, and the baking powder provides a light, fluffy texture.

This 5•ingredient recipe is a great option for those with diverticulitis, as it is low in fiber and gentle on the digestive system. Enjoy this simple, nourishing cake as a treat or snack.

45. Banana Muffins:
Bananas, flour, sugar, eggs, baking powder.

Ingredients:

1. Ripe bananas, mashed
2. Gluten•free flour (such as almond or oat flour)
3. Honey (or maple syrup)
4. Eggs
5. Baking powder

Instructions:

1. Preheat your oven to 350°F (175°C). Grease a 12•cup muffin tin or line with paper liners.

2. In a medium bowl, mash the ripe bananas until smooth.

3. Add the gluten•free flour, honey (or maple syrup), eggs, and baking powder to the mashed bananas. Stir until just combined, being careful not to overmix.

4. Scoop the batter evenly into the prepared muffin cups, filling them about 3/4 full.

5. Bake for 18•22 minutes, or until a toothpick inserted into the center comes out clean.

6. Allow the muffins to cool in the tin for 5 minutes before transferring to a wire rack to cool completely.

These banana muffins are a gentle, diverticulitis•friendly treat. The ripe bananas provide natural sweetness and moisture, while the gluten•free flour and honey (or maple syrup) create a tender, easy•to•digest muffin. The eggs help bind the ingredients together, and the baking powder gives the muffins a light, fluffy texture.

This 5•ingredient recipe is a great option for those with diverticulitis, as it is low in fiber and gentle on the digestive system. Enjoy these nourishing banana muffins as a snack or breakfast.

46. Greek Yogurt with Honey: Greek yogurt, honey.

Ingredients:

1. Plain Greek yogurt
2. Honey
3. Cinnamon
4. Vanilla extract
5. Sliced almonds (optional)

Instructions:

1. Scoop the desired amount of plain Greek yogurt into a bowl.

2. Drizzle honey over the yogurt, to taste.

3. Sprinkle a pinch of cinnamon over the top.

4. Add a splash of vanilla extract and stir to combine.

5. Top with a few sliced almonds, if desired.

This simple, 5•ingredient recipe is gentle on the digestive system for those with diverticulitis. The Greek yogurt provides a good source of protein and probiotics, while the honey adds natural sweetness without being too harsh on the gut. The cinnamon and vanilla extract provide additional flavor without irritating the digestive tract.

The optional sliced almonds add a crunchy texture and healthy fats, which can be included if tolerated. This Greek yogurt with honey dish makes for a nourishing and soothing snack or light meal for those with diverticulitis.

47. Oatmeal Cookies:
Oats, flour, sugar, eggs, butter.

Ingredients:

1. Rolled oats
2. Gluten•free flour (such as almond or oat flour)
3. Honey (or maple syrup)
4. Eggs
5. Coconut oil (or unsalted butter)

Instructions:

1. Preheat your oven to 350°F (175°C). Line a baking sheet with parchment paper.

2. In a medium bowl, mix together the rolled oats and gluten•free flour.

3. In a separate bowl, whisk the honey (or maple syrup), eggs, and melted coconut oil (or unsalted butter) until well combined.

4. Gently fold the wet ingredients into the dry ingredients until just combined, being careful not to overmix.

5. Scoop the dough by the tablespoonful onto the prepared baking sheet, spacing them about 2 inches apart.

6. Bake for 12•15 minutes, or until the cookies are lightly golden around the edges.

7. Allow the cookies to cool on the baking sheet for 5 minutes before transferring to a wire rack to cool completely.

These oatmeal cookies are a gentle, diverticulitis•friendly treat. The rolled oats provide a source of fiber, while the gluten•free flour and honey (or maple syrup) create a tender, easy•to•digest cookie. The eggs help bind the ingredients together, and the coconut oil (or unsalted butter) adds richness without being too harsh on the digestive system.

This 5•ingredient recipe is a great option for those with diverticulitis, as it is low in fiber and gentle on the gut. Enjoy these nourishing oatmeal cookies as a snack or light dessert.

48. Smoothie Popsicles:
Banana, yogurt, berries, honey.

Ingredients:

1. Ripe banana, frozen
2. Plain Greek yogurt
3. Frozen berries (such as blueberries or raspberries)
4. Honey (or maple syrup)
5. Unsweetened almond milk (optional)

Instructions:

1. In a blender, combine the frozen banana, Greek yogurt, frozen berries, and honey (or maple syrup). Blend until smooth and creamy.

2. If the mixture is too thick, add a splash of unsweetened almond milk and blend again until you reach your desired consistency.

3. Carefully pour the smoothie mixture into popsicle molds, leaving a small amount of space at the top for expansion.

4. Insert popsicle sticks and freeze for at least 4 hours, or until completely set.

5. To remove the popsicles, run the molds under warm water for a few seconds before gently pulling them out.

These smoothie popsicles are a gentle, diverticulitis•friendly treat. The banana and Greek yogurt provide a creamy base, while the frozen berries add natural sweetness and antioxidants. The honey (or maple syrup) enhances the flavor without being too harsh on the digestive system.

The optional almond milk can be added to thin out the mixture if needed, making it easier to pour into the popsicle molds. This 5•ingredient recipe is a great way to enjoy a refreshing, nourishing snack that is gentle on the gut.

49. Baked Apples: Apples, cinnamon, sugar, butter.

Ingredients:

1. Apples (such as Gala or Fuji), cored and halved
2. Cinnamon
3. Honey (or maple syrup)
4. Unsweetened almond milk (or dairy milk)
5. Walnuts, chopped (optional)

Instructions:

1. Preheat your oven to 375°F (190°C). Grease a baking dish or line it with parchment paper.

2. Place the apple halves, cut•side up, in the prepared baking dish.

3. Sprinkle the apples with a generous amount of cinnamon.

4. Drizzle the apples with honey (or maple syrup) and a splash of almond milk (or dairy milk).

5. Bake for 20•25 minutes, or until the apples are tender when pierced with a fork.

6. If desired, sprinkle the baked apples with chopped walnuts before serving.

These baked apples are a gentle, diverticulitis•friendly dessert or snack. The apples provide natural sweetness and fiber, while the cinnamon and honey (or maple syrup) add flavor without being too harsh on the digestive system. The optional walnuts provide a crunchy texture and healthy fats.

The almond milk (or dairy milk) helps keep the apples moist during baking, creating a soft, easy•to•digest texture. This 5•ingredient recipe is a great way to enjoy a comforting, nourishing treat that is gentle on the gut.

50. Fruit Sorbet: Berries, sugar, lemon juice, water.

Ingredients:

1. Frozen berries (such as raspberries, blackberries, or blueberries)
2. Honey (or maple syrup)
3. Lemon juice
4. Water
5. Mint leaves (optional)

Instructions:

1. In a high•powered blender or food processor, combine the frozen berries, honey (or maple syrup), lemon juice, and water.

2. Blend the mixture until smooth and creamy, scraping down the sides as needed.

3. Taste and adjust sweetener or lemon juice as desired.

4. Transfer the sorbet mixture to a freezer•safe container and freeze for 2•3 hours, stirring every 30 minutes, until the sorbet reaches your desired consistency.

5. Serve the sorbet immediately, garnished with fresh mint leaves if desired.

This fruit sorbet is a gentle, diverticulitis•friendly dessert. The frozen berries provide the base, while the honey (or maple syrup) adds sweetness without being too harsh on the digestive system. The lemon juice provides a refreshing tartness, and the water helps create a smooth, scoopable texture.

The optional mint leaves add a subtle flavor boost without irritating the gut. This 5•ingredient sorbet is a great way to enjoy a cool, nourishing treat that is gentle on the digestive system.

51. Chicken Noodle Soup:
Chicken breast, noodles, carrots, celery, broth.

Ingredients:

1. Boneless, skinless chicken breasts
2. Gluten•free noodles (such as rice or quinoa noodles)
3. Carrots, peeled and sliced
4. Celery, sliced
5. Low•sodium chicken broth

Instructions:

1. In a large pot, place the chicken breasts and cover with the chicken broth.

2. Bring the broth to a boil, then reduce the heat and simmer for 15•20 minutes, or until the chicken is cooked through.

3. Remove the chicken from the pot and shred or dice it.

4. Return the shredded chicken to the pot and add the sliced carrots and celery.

5. Bring the soup back to a simmer and add the gluten•free noodles. Cook for an additional 8•10 minutes, or until the noodles are tender.

6. Serve the chicken noodle soup hot.

This 5•ingredient chicken noodle soup is a gentle, diverticulitis•friendly option. The chicken provides a lean protein source, while the gluten•free noodles, carrots, and celery are easy to digest. The low•sodium chicken broth helps to keep the soup light and soothing on the digestive system.

This simple soup is a great choice for those with diverticulitis, as it is low in fiber and easy on the gut. Adjust the cooking time for the noodles as needed to achieve your desired texture.

52. Butternut Squash Soup:
Butternut squash, broth, cream, salt, pepper.

Ingredients:

1. Butternut squash, peeled, seeded, and cubed
2. Unsweetened almond milk (or dairy milk)
3. Vegetable or chicken broth
4. Salt
5. Pepper

Instructions:

1. In a large pot or Dutch oven, combine the cubed butternut squash and broth.

2. Bring the mixture to a boil, then reduce the heat and simmer for 20•25 minutes, or until the squash is very soft.

3. Remove the pot from the heat and use an immersion blender to puree the soup until smooth.

4. Stir in the almond milk (or dairy milk) and season with salt and pepper to taste.

5. Reheat the soup gently over low heat, stirring occasionally, until heated through.

This 5•ingredient butternut squash soup is a gentle, diverticulitis•friendly option. The butternut squash provides a creamy, nutrient•dense base, while the almond milk (or dairy milk) adds creaminess without being too heavy on the digestive system. The broth helps to thin out the soup and provide a soothing, comforting texture.

The simple seasoning of salt and pepper allows the natural sweetness of the squash to shine through without overwhelming the gut. This soup is an easy, nourishing option for those with diverticulitis.

53. Tomato Soup: Tomatoes, broth, cream, salt, basil.

Ingredients:

1. Canned diced tomatoes (or fresh tomatoes, peeled and diced)
2. Unsweetened almond milk (or dairy milk)
3. Vegetable or chicken broth
4. Salt
5. Fresh basil leaves (optional)

Instructions:

1. In a large saucepan or pot, combine the diced tomatoes and broth.

2. Bring the mixture to a simmer over medium heat, then reduce the heat and let it simmer for 10•15 minutes, stirring occasionally.

3. Remove the pot from the heat and use an immersion blender to puree the soup until smooth.

4. Stir in the almond milk (or dairy milk) and season with salt to taste.

5. Reheat the soup gently over low heat, stirring occasionally, until heated through.

6. Serve the tomato soup warm, garnished with fresh basil leaves if desired.

This 5•ingredient tomato soup is a gentle, diverticulitis•friendly option. The canned or fresh tomatoes provide the base, while the almond milk (or dairy milk) adds creaminess without being too heavy on the digestive system. The broth helps to thin out the soup and provide a soothing, comforting texture.

The simple seasoning of salt allows the natural flavors of the tomatoes to shine through without overwhelming the gut. The optional fresh basil leaves add a touch of flavor without being too harsh. This soup is an easy, nourishing option for those with diverticulitis.

54. Broccoli Cheddar Soup:
Broccoli, cheddar cheese, milk, butter, salt.

Ingredients:

1. Broccoli florets
2. Unsweetened almond milk (or dairy milk)
3. Grated cheddar cheese (or dairy•free cheese alternative)
4. Olive oil (or unsalted butter)
5. Salt

Instructions:

1. In a large pot, sauté the broccoli florets in the olive oil (or melt the butter) over medium heat until tender, about 5•7 minutes.

2. Add the almond milk (or dairy milk) to the pot and bring the mixture to a simmer.

3. Reduce the heat to low and gradually stir in the grated cheddar cheese (or dairy•free cheese alternative) until it's melted and the soup is creamy.

4. Season the soup with salt to taste.

5. Serve the broccoli cheddar soup warm.

This 5•ingredient broccoli cheddar soup is a gentle, diverticulitis•friendly option. The broccoli provides fiber and nutrients, while the almond milk (or dairy milk) and cheese create a creamy texture without being too heavy on the digestive system.

The olive oil (or unsalted butter) adds a touch of richness, and the simple seasoning of salt allows the natural flavors to shine through without overwhelming the gut. This soup is an easy, nourishing option for those with diverticulitis.

55. Pumpkin Soup:
Pumpkin, broth, cream, salt, pepper.

Ingredients:

1. Canned pumpkin puree (or roasted and mashed pumpkin)
2. Unsweetened almond milk (or dairy milk)
3. Vegetable or chicken broth
4. Salt
5. Ground black pepper

Instructions:

1. In a large saucepan or pot, combine the pumpkin puree and broth.

2. Bring the mixture to a simmer over medium heat, then reduce the heat and let it simmer for 10•15 minutes, stirring occasionally.

3. Remove the pot from the heat and use an immersion blender to puree the soup until smooth.

4. Stir in the almond milk (or dairy milk) and season with salt and ground black pepper to taste.

5. Reheat the soup gently over low heat, stirring occasionally, until heated through.

This 5•ingredient pumpkin soup is a gentle, diverticulitis•friendly option. The pumpkin puree provides a creamy, nutrient•dense base, while the almond milk (or dairy milk) adds creaminess without being too heavy on the digestive system. The broth helps to thin out the soup and provide a soothing, comforting texture.

The simple seasoning of salt and ground black pepper allows the natural flavors of the pumpkin to shine through without overwhelming the gut. This soup is an easy, nourishing option for those with diverticulitis.

56. Carrot Ginger Soup:
Carrots, ginger, broth, cream, salt.

Ingredients:

1. Carrots, peeled and sliced
2. Fresh ginger, peeled and grated
3. Unsweetened almond milk (or dairy milk)
4. Vegetable or chicken broth
5. Salt

Instructions:

1. In a large pot, combine the sliced carrots, grated ginger, and broth.

2. Bring the mixture to a boil, then reduce the heat and simmer for 20•25 minutes, or until the carrots are very soft.

3. Remove the pot from the heat and use an immersion blender to puree the soup until smooth.

4. Stir in the almond milk (or dairy milk) and season with salt to taste.

5. Reheat the soup gently over low heat, stirring occasionally, until heated through.

This 5•ingredient carrot ginger soup is a gentle, diverticulitis•friendly option. The carrots provide a natural sweetness and fiber, while the ginger adds a subtle warmth and anti•inflammatory properties. The almond milk (or dairy milk) adds creaminess without being too heavy on the digestive system.

The simple seasoning of salt allows the natural flavors to shine through without overwhelming the gut. This soup is an easy, nourishing option for those with diverticulitis, as it is low in fiber and gentle on the digestive system.

57. Potato Leek Soup:
Potatoes, leeks, broth, cream, salt.

Ingredients:

1. Potatoes, peeled and diced
2. Leeks, sliced (white and light green parts only)
3. Unsweetened almond milk (or dairy milk)
4. Vegetable or chicken broth
5. Salt

Instructions:

1. In a large pot, combine the diced potatoes, sliced leeks, and broth.

2. Bring the mixture to a boil, then reduce the heat and simmer for 20•25 minutes, or until the potatoes are very soft.

3. Remove the pot from the heat and use an immersion blender to puree the soup until smooth.

4. Stir in the almond milk (or dairy milk) and season with salt to taste.

5. Reheat the soup gently over low heat, stirring occasionally, until heated through.

This 5•ingredient potato leek soup is a gentle, diverticulitis•friendly option. The potatoes provide a creamy base, while the leeks add a subtle onion•like flavor without being too harsh on the digestive system. The almond milk (or dairy milk) adds creaminess without being too heavy.

The simple seasoning of salt allows the natural flavors to shine through without overwhelming the gut. This soup is an easy, nourishing option for those with diverticulitis, as it is low in fiber and gentle on the digestive system.

58. Cauliflower Soup:
Cauliflower, broth, cream, salt, pepper.

Ingredients:

1. Cauliflower florets
2. Unsweetened almond milk (or dairy milk)
3. Vegetable or chicken broth
4. Salt
5. Ground black pepper

Instructions:

1. In a large pot, combine the cauliflower florets and broth.

2. Bring the mixture to a boil, then reduce the heat and simmer for 15•20 minutes, or until the cauliflower is very soft.

3. Remove the pot from the heat and use an immersion blender to puree the soup until smooth.

4. Stir in the almond milk (or dairy milk) and season with salt and ground black pepper to taste.

5. Reheat the soup gently over low heat, stirring occasionally, until heated through.

This 5•ingredient cauliflower soup is a gentle, diverticulitis•friendly option. The cauliflower provides a creamy, nutrient•dense base, while the almond milk (or dairy milk) adds creaminess without being too heavy on the digestive system. The broth helps to thin out the soup and provide a soothing, comforting texture.

The simple seasoning of salt and ground black pepper allows the natural flavors of the cauliflower to shine through without overwhelming the gut. This soup is an easy, nourishing option for those with diverticulitis, as it is low in fiber and gentle on the digestive system.

59. Zucchini Soup:
Zucchini, broth, cream, salt, pepper.

Ingredients:

1. Zucchini, diced
2. Unsweetened almond milk (or dairy milk)
3. Vegetable or chicken broth
4. Salt
5. Ground black pepper

Instructions:

1. In a large pot, combine the diced zucchini and broth.

2. Bring the mixture to a boil, then reduce the heat and simmer for 15•20 minutes, or until the zucchini is very soft.

3. Remove the pot from the heat and use an immersion blender to puree the soup until smooth.

4. Stir in the almond milk (or dairy milk) and season with salt and ground black pepper to taste.

5. Reheat the soup gently over low heat, stirring occasionally, until heated through.

This 5•ingredient zucchini soup is a gentle, diverticulitis•friendly option. The zucchini provides a creamy, nutrient•dense base, while the almond milk (or dairy milk) adds creaminess without being too heavy on the digestive system. The broth helps to thin out the soup and provide a soothing, comforting texture.

The simple seasoning of salt and ground black pepper allows the natural flavors of the zucchini to shine through without overwhelming the gut. This soup is an easy, nourishing option for those with diverticulitis, as it is low in fiber and gentle on the digestive system.

60. Celery Soup: Celery, broth, cream, salt, pepper.

Ingredients:

1. Celery, chopped
2. Unsweetened almond milk (or dairy milk)
3. Vegetable or chicken broth
4. Salt
5. Ground black pepper

Instructions:

1. In a large pot, combine the chopped celery and broth.

2. Bring the mixture to a boil, then reduce the heat and simmer for 15•20 minutes, or until the celery is very soft.

3. Remove the pot from the heat and use an immersion blender to puree the soup until smooth.

4. Stir in the almond milk (or dairy milk) and season with salt and ground black pepper to taste.

5. Reheat the soup gently over low heat, stirring occasionally, until heated through.

This 5•ingredient celery soup is a gentle, diverticulitis•friendly option. The celery provides a mild, nutrient•dense base, while the almond milk (or dairy milk) adds creaminess without being too heavy on the digestive system. The broth helps to thin out the soup and provide a soothing, comforting texture.

The simple seasoning of salt and ground black pepper allows the natural flavors of the celery to shine through without overwhelming the gut. This soup is an easy, nourishing option for those with diverticulitis, as it is low in fiber and gentle on the digestive system.

61. Vegetable Stir•Fry:
Carrots, broccoli, bell peppers, soy sauce, olive oil.

Ingredients:

1. Carrots, sliced
2. Broccoli florets
3. Bell peppers, sliced
4. Coconut aminos (or low•sodium soy sauce)
5. Olive oil

Instructions:

1. In a large skillet or wok, heat the olive oil over medium•high heat.

2. Add the sliced carrots, broccoli florets, and bell pepper slices. Stir•fry for 5•7 minutes, or until the vegetables are tender•crisp.

3. Reduce the heat to low and add the coconut aminos (or low•sodium soy sauce). Stir to coat the vegetables evenly.

4. Cook for an additional 2•3 minutes, allowing the sauce to thicken slightly.

5. Serve the vegetable stir•fry immediately.

This 5•ingredient vegetable stir•fry is a gentle, diverticulitis•friendly option. The carrots, broccoli, and bell peppers provide a variety of vitamins, minerals, and fiber, while the coconut aminos (or low•sodium soy sauce) add flavor without being too harsh on the digestive system.

The olive oil helps to sauté the vegetables without adding too much fat. This simple stir•fry is easy to digest and gentle on the gut, making it a great choice for those with diverticulitis.

62. Stuffed Peppers:
Bell peppers, rice, tomato sauce, cheese, salt.

Ingredients:

1. Bell peppers, halved and seeded
2. Cooked white rice
3. Canned diced tomatoes or tomato sauce
4. Shredded mozzarella cheese (or dairy•free cheese alternative)
5. Salt

Instructions:

1. Preheat your oven to 375°F (190°C).

2. Place the bell pepper halves in a baking dish, cut•side up.

3. In a bowl, mix together the cooked white rice, canned diced tomatoes (or tomato sauce), and a pinch of salt.

4. Spoon the rice mixture into the bell pepper halves, filling them evenly.

5. Top the stuffed peppers with the shredded mozzarella cheese (or dairy•free cheese alternative).

6. Bake for 25•30 minutes, or until the peppers are tender and the cheese is melted and bubbly.

This 5•ingredient stuffed peppers recipe is a gentle, diverticulitis•friendly option. The bell peppers provide a low•fiber, easy•to•digest vegetable base, while the white rice and tomato sauce create a soothing, comforting filling. The mozzarella cheese (or dairy•free alternative) adds a touch of creaminess without being too heavy on the digestive system.

The simple seasoning of salt allows the natural flavors to shine through without overwhelming the gut. This dish is a great way to enjoy a nourishing, diverticulitis•friendly meal.

63. Baked Potatoes:
Potatoes, butter, sour cream, salt, pepper.

Ingredients:

1. Russet potatoes
2. Unsweetened almond milk (or dairy milk)
3. Olive oil or avocado oil
4. Salt
5. Ground black pepper

Instructions:

1. Preheat your oven to 400°F (200°C).

2. Scrub the potatoes and prick them several times with a fork.

3. Rub the potatoes with a small amount of olive oil or avocado oil and sprinkle with salt.

4. Bake the potatoes directly on the oven rack for 50•60 minutes, or until they are tender when pierced with a fork.

5. Remove the potatoes from the oven and let them cool for a few minutes.

6. Slice the potatoes open and fluff the insides with a fork.

7. Drizzle the potatoes with a small amount of almond milk (or dairy milk) and season with salt and ground black pepper to taste.

This 5•ingredient baked potato recipe is a gentle, diverticulitis•friendly option. The potatoes provide a source of carbohydrates and potassium, while the almond milk (or dairy milk) adds a creamy texture without being too heavy on the digestive system.

The simple seasoning of salt and ground black pepper allows the natural flavors to shine through without overwhelming the gut. This dish is a great way to enjoy a comforting, nourishing meal that is gentle on the digestive system.

64. Spinach Omelet:
Eggs, spinach, cheese, salt, pepper.

Ingredients:

1. Eggs
2. Fresh spinach, chopped
3. Shredded mozzarella cheese (or dairy•free cheese alternative)
4. Salt
5. Ground black pepper

Instructions:

1. Crack the eggs into a bowl and whisk them lightly with a fork. Season with a pinch of salt and ground black pepper.

2. In a nonstick skillet, sauté the chopped spinach over medium heat until it's wilted, about 2•3 minutes.

3. Pour the whisked eggs over the spinach and let the bottom set for 1•2 minutes.

4. Sprinkle the shredded mozzarella cheese (or dairy•free cheese alternative) over the top of the eggs.

5. Fold the omelet in half and slide it onto a plate. Serve immediately.

This 5•ingredient spinach omelet is a gentle, diverticulitis•friendly option. The eggs provide a good source of protein, while the spinach adds fiber and nutrients without being too harsh on the digestive system. The mozzarella cheese (or dairy•free alternative) adds a creamy texture without being too heavy.

The simple seasoning of salt and ground black pepper allows the natural flavors to shine through without overwhelming the gut. This omelet is a great way to enjoy a nourishing, easy•to•digest meal that is gentle on the digestive system.

65. Tomato Basil Pasta:
Pasta, tomatoes, basil, olive oil, garlic.

Ingredients:

1. Gluten•free pasta (such as brown rice or quinoa pasta)
2. Canned diced tomatoes
3. Fresh basil leaves
4. Olive oil
5. Garlic, minced

Instructions:

1. Cook the gluten•free pasta according to the package instructions. Drain and set aside.

2. In a large skillet, heat the olive oil over medium heat. Add the minced garlic and sauté for 1•2 minutes, until fragrant.

3. Add the canned diced tomatoes (with their juices) to the skillet. Bring the mixture to a simmer and let it cook for 5•7 minutes, stirring occasionally, until the sauce has thickened slightly.

4. Remove the skillet from the heat and stir in the cooked pasta and fresh basil leaves until well combined.

5. Serve the tomato basil pasta warm.

This 5•ingredient tomato basil pasta is a gentle, diverticulitis•friendly option. The gluten•free pasta provides a source of carbohydrates without being too harsh on the digestive system. The canned diced tomatoes and fresh basil leaves add flavor and nutrients, while the olive oil and garlic provide a subtle seasoning.

This simple pasta dish is easy to digest and gentle on the gut, making it a great choice for those with diverticulitis. Adjust the amount of garlic or basil to your personal taste preferences.

66. Vegetable Soup:
Carrots, celery, potatoes, broth, salt.

Ingredients:

1. Carrots, peeled and sliced
2. Celery, sliced
3. Potatoes, peeled and diced
4. Vegetable or chicken broth
5. Salt

Instructions:

1. In a large pot, combine the sliced carrots, celery, and diced potatoes.

2. Pour in the vegetable or chicken broth, making sure the vegetables are fully submerged.

3. Bring the soup to a boil over medium·high heat, then reduce the heat and let it simmer for 20·25 minutes, or until the vegetables are tender.

4. Season the soup with salt to taste.

5. Serve the vegetable soup warm.

This 5·ingredient vegetable soup is a gentle, diverticulitis·friendly option. The carrots, celery, and potatoes provide a variety of nutrients without being too high in fiber. The broth creates a soothing, comforting base for the soup.

The simple seasoning of salt allows the natural flavors of the vegetables to shine through without overwhelming the gut. This soup is an easy, nourishing option for those with diverticulitis, as it is low in fiber and gentle on the digestive system.

You can adjust the cooking time for the vegetables to your desired texture. This soup can be a great way to incorporate more vegetables into your diet while being gentle on the digestive system.

67. Caprese Salad: Tomatoes, mozzarella, basil, olive oil, balsamic vinegar.

Ingredients:

1. Tomatoes, sliced
2. Fresh mozzarella cheese, sliced
3. Fresh basil leaves
4. Olive oil
5. Balsamic glaze (or reduced balsamic vinegar)

Instructions:

1. Arrange the sliced tomatoes and mozzarella cheese on a serving plate or platter.

2. Gently tear or chiffonade the fresh basil leaves and sprinkle them over the tomatoes and cheese.

3. Drizzle the salad with a high•quality olive oil.

4. Finish the dish by drizzling a small amount of balsamic glaze (or reduced balsamic vinegar) over the top.

5. Season with a pinch of salt, if desired.

This 5•ingredient Caprese salad is a gentle, diverticulitis•friendly option. The tomatoes and mozzarella provide a balance of nutrients without being too high in fiber, while the fresh basil adds flavor without irritating the digestive system.

The olive oil and balsamic glaze (or reduced vinegar) provide a simple dressing that is easy to digest. This salad is a refreshing and nourishing choice for those with diverticulitis, as it is low in fiber and gentle on the gut.

You can adjust the amounts of each ingredient to suit your personal taste preferences. Enjoy this simple, yet flavorful Caprese salad as a light meal or side dish.

68. Creamed Spinach:
Spinach, cream, butter, salt, pepper.

Ingredients:

1. Fresh spinach, washed and chopped
2. Unsweetened almond milk (or dairy milk)
3. Unsalted butter
4. Salt
5. Ground black pepper

Instructions:

1. In a large skillet or saucepan, melt the butter over medium heat.

2. Add the chopped spinach to the skillet and sauté for 2•3 minutes, until the spinach is wilted.

3. Slowly pour in the almond milk (or dairy milk) and stir to combine.

4. Reduce the heat to low and let the mixture simmer, stirring occasionally, until the sauce has thickened slightly, about 5•7 minutes.

5. Season the creamed spinach with salt and ground black pepper to taste.

6. Serve the creamed spinach warm.

This 5•ingredient creamed spinach is a gentle, diverticulitis•friendly option. The spinach provides a good source of nutrients without being too high in fiber, while the almond milk (or dairy milk) and butter create a creamy, soothing texture.

The simple seasoning of salt and ground black pepper allows the natural flavors to shine through without overwhelming the gut. This dish is an easy, nourishing way to incorporate more leafy greens into your diet while being gentle on the digestive system.

You can adjust the amount of milk and butter to achieve your desired consistency. Enjoy this creamed spinach as a side dish or light meal.

69. Eggplant Parmesan: Eggplant, marinara sauce, mozzarella, parmesan, breadcrumbs.

Ingredients:

- 1 large eggplant, sliced into 1/2•inch thick rounds
- 1 cup marinara sauce
- 1 cup shredded mozzarella cheese
- 1/2 cup grated parmesan cheese
- 1 cup breadcrumbs

Instructions:

1. Preheat oven to 375°F. Grease a baking sheet or casserole dish.

2. Dip the eggplant slices in the marinara sauce, coating both sides.

3. Arrange the eggplant slices in a single layer on the prepared baking sheet or dish.

4. Sprinkle the mozzarella and parmesan cheeses evenly over the eggplant.

5. Top with the breadcrumbs.

6. Bake for 25•30 minutes, until the eggplant is tender and the cheese is melted and bubbly.

7. Let cool for 5 minutes before serving.

Enjoy your homemade Eggplant Parmesan!

70. Vegetable Quiche: Eggs, spinach, cheese, milk, salt.

Ingredients:

• 6 eggs
• 1 cup fresh spinach, chopped
• 1 cup shredded cheese (such as cheddar or mozzarella)
• 1 cup milk
• 1/2 teaspoon salt

Instructions:

1. Preheat oven to 375°F. Grease a 9•inch pie dish.

2. In a large bowl, whisk together the eggs, milk, and salt until well combined.

3. Stir in the chopped spinach and shredded cheese.

4. Pour the egg mixture into the prepared pie dish.

5. Bake for 35•40 minutes, until the center is set and the top is lightly golden.

6. Allow the quiche to cool for 5•10 minutes before slicing and serving.

This quiche recipe keeps things simple with just 5 main ingredients • eggs, spinach, cheese, milk, and salt. The spinach provides fiber and nutrients, while the cheese and eggs create a protein•rich filling. The milk helps bind everything together. This makes for a nutritious and easy•to•digest meal that is suitable for those following a diverticulitis•friendly diet.

71. Grilled Shrimp:
Shrimp, olive oil, lemon, garlic, salt.

Ingredients:

• 1 lb large shrimp, peeled and deveined
• 2 tablespoons olive oil
• 1 tablespoon lemon juice
• 2 cloves garlic, minced
• 1/2 teaspoon salt

Instructions:

1. In a large bowl, combine the shrimp, olive oil, lemon juice, minced garlic, and salt. Toss to coat the shrimp evenly.

2. Preheat grill or grill pan to medium•high heat.

3. Thread the shrimp onto skewers, leaving a little space between each one.

4. Grill the shrimp for 2•3 minutes per side, until they are opaque and cooked through.

5. Serve the grilled shrimp immediately, squeezing extra lemon juice over the top if desired.

This simple grilled shrimp recipe uses just 5 main ingredients • shrimp, olive oil, lemon, garlic, and salt. The lemon and garlic add flavor without being too heavy, while the olive oil helps the shrimp stay moist during grilling. This makes for a light, easy•to•digest meal that is suitable for those following a diverticulitis•friendly diet.

72. Baked Salmon:
Salmon, lemon, olive oil, salt, dill.

Ingredients:

• 4 salmon fillets (about 1 lb total)
• 2 tablespoons olive oil
• 1 tablespoon lemon juice
• 1 teaspoon dried dill
• 1/2 teaspoon salt

Instructions:

1. Preheat your oven to 400°F. Line a baking sheet with parchment paper or foil.

2. Place the salmon fillets on the prepared baking sheet.

3. In a small bowl, whisk together the olive oil, lemon juice, dried dill, and salt.

4. Drizzle the olive oil mixture evenly over the top of the salmon fillets, making sure to coat them completely.

5. Bake the salmon for 12•15 minutes, or until it flakes easily with a fork and is cooked through.

6. Serve the baked salmon immediately, garnished with extra lemon wedges if desired.

This simple baked salmon recipe uses just 5 main ingredients • salmon, olive oil, lemon, dill, and salt. The lemon and dill add flavor without being too heavy, while the olive oil helps keep the salmon moist during baking. This makes for a light, easy•to•digest meal that is suitable for those following a diverticulitis•friendly diet.

73. Tuna Salad: Canned tuna, mayonnaise, salt, pepper, lemon juice.

Ingredients:

• 2 (5 oz) cans of tuna, drained
• 1/4 cup mayonnaise
• 1 tablespoon lemon juice
• 1/4 teaspoon salt
• 1/4 teaspoon ground black pepper

Instructions:

1. In a medium bowl, combine the drained tuna, mayonnaise, lemon juice, salt, and black pepper.

2. Mix everything together until the tuna is well coated and the ingredients are evenly distributed.

3. Taste and adjust seasoning as needed, adding more salt, pepper, or lemon juice to your preference.

4. Serve the tuna salad on its own, on top of lettuce or greens, or as a sandwich filling.

This tuna salad recipe keeps things simple with just 5 main ingredients • canned tuna, mayonnaise, lemon juice, salt, and pepper. The mayonnaise provides creaminess, while the lemon juice and seasoning add flavor without being too heavy. This makes for a light, easy•to•digest meal that is suitable for those following a diverticulitis•friendly diet.

74. Fish Tacos:
White fish, tortillas, lime, cabbage, salsa.

Ingredients:

• 1 lb white fish fillets (such as tilapia, cod, or halibut), cut into 1•inch pieces
• 8 small corn or flour tortillas
• 1 lime, cut into wedges
• 2 cups shredded cabbage
• 1/2 cup salsa

Instructions:

1. Preheat your oven to 400°F. Line a baking sheet with parchment paper.

2. Place the fish pieces on the prepared baking sheet. Bake for 10•12 minutes, until the fish is opaque and flakes easily with a fork.

3. Warm the tortillas according to package instructions, either in the oven, on the stovetop, or in the microwave.

4. To assemble the tacos, place a portion of the baked fish into each tortilla. Top with shredded cabbage and a spoonful of salsa.

5. Serve the fish tacos immediately, with lime wedges on the side for squeezing over the top.

This fish taco recipe uses just 5 main ingredients • white fish, tortillas, lime, cabbage, and salsa. The baked fish provides a lean protein, while the cabbage and salsa add freshness and flavor without being too heavy. The lime adds a bright, acidic note to balance the dish. This makes for a light, easy•to•digest meal that is suitable for those following a diverticulitis•friendly diet.

75. Shrimp Scampi:
Shrimp, garlic, butter, lemon, parsley.

Ingredients:

• 1 lb large shrimp, peeled and deveined
• 3 cloves garlic, minced
• 4 tablespoons unsalted butter
• 1 tablespoon lemon juice
• 2 tablespoons chopped fresh parsley

Instructions:

1. In a large skillet, melt the butter over medium heat. Add the minced garlic and cook for 1•2 minutes, until fragrant.

2. Add the shrimp to the skillet and cook for 2•3 minutes per side, until the shrimp are pink and opaque.

3. Remove the skillet from the heat and stir in the lemon juice and chopped parsley. Toss to coat the shrimp evenly.

4. Serve the shrimp scampi immediately, with the garlic•butter sauce spooned over the top.

This shrimp scampi recipe uses just 5 main ingredients • shrimp, garlic, butter, lemon, and parsley. The butter and lemon create a rich, flavorful sauce, while the parsley adds a fresh, herbal note. This makes for a simple, yet elegant dish that is suitable for those following a diverticulitis•friendly diet.

76. Crab Cakes: Crab meat, breadcrumbs, egg, mayonnaise, lemon juice.

Ingredients:

• 1 lb lump crab meat, picked over for shells
• 1/2 cup panko breadcrumbs
• 1 egg, lightly beaten
• 2 tablespoons mayonnaise
• 1 tablespoon lemon juice

Instructions:

1. In a large bowl, gently mix together the crab meat, panko breadcrumbs, egg, mayonnaise, and lemon juice until just combined. Be careful not to overmix.

2. Form the mixture into 4•6 crab cakes, about 1/2 inch thick.

3. Heat a large skillet over medium heat and add 1•2 tablespoons of olive oil or butter.

4. Carefully add the crab cakes to the hot skillet and cook for 3•4 minutes per side, until golden brown.

5. Serve the crab cakes immediately, with extra lemon wedges on the side.

This crab cake recipe uses just 5 main ingredients • crab meat, panko breadcrumbs, egg, mayonnaise, and lemon juice. The mayonnaise and egg help bind the crab cakes together, while the lemon juice adds a bright, acidic note. This makes for a light, flavorful dish that is suitable for those following a diverticulitis•friendly diet.

77. Baked Cod:
Cod fillet, lemon, olive oil, garlic, salt.

Ingredients:

- 1 lb cod fillets
- 2 tablespoons olive oil
- 1 tablespoon lemon juice
- 2 cloves garlic, minced
- 1/2 teaspoon salt

Instructions:

1. Preheat your oven to 400°F. Grease a baking dish or line a baking sheet with parchment paper.

2. Place the cod fillets in the prepared baking dish or on the baking sheet.

3. In a small bowl, whisk together the olive oil, lemon juice, minced garlic, and salt.

4. Drizzle the olive oil mixture over the top of the cod fillets, making sure to evenly coat them.

5. Bake the cod for 12•15 minutes, or until it flakes easily with a fork and is opaque throughout.

6. Serve the baked cod immediately, garnished with extra lemon wedges if desired.

This baked cod recipe uses just 5 main ingredients • cod, olive oil, lemon, garlic, and salt. The olive oil and lemon juice help keep the cod moist and add flavor, while the garlic and salt provide seasoning. This makes for a simple, yet delicious dish that is suitable for those following a diverticulitis•friendly diet.

78. Seared Scallops:
Scallops, butter, garlic, lemon, parsley.

Ingredients:

• 1 lb sea scallops, patted dry
• 2 tablespoons unsalted butter
• 2 cloves garlic, minced
• 1 tablespoon lemon juice
• 2 tablespoons chopped fresh parsley

Instructions:

1. Heat a large skillet over high heat. Add the butter and let it melt and start to sizzle.

2. Working in batches if needed, add the scallops to the hot skillet in a single layer. Sear for 2•3 minutes per side, until they develop a nice golden•brown crust.

3. Remove the scallops from the skillet and set them aside on a plate.

4. Reduce the heat to medium•low and add the minced garlic to the skillet. Cook for 1 minute, stirring constantly, until fragrant.

5. Remove the skillet from the heat and stir in the lemon juice and chopped parsley.

6. Return the seared scallops to the skillet and toss to coat them in the garlic•lemon•parsley sauce.

7. Serve the seared scallops immediately, while hot.

This seared scallops recipe uses just 5 main ingredients • scallops, butter, garlic, lemon, and parsley. The butter and lemon create a simple, yet flavorful sauce, while the parsley adds a fresh, herbal note. This makes for a light, easy•to•digest meal that is suitable for those following a diverticulitis•friendly diet.

79. Clam Chowder:
Clams, potatoes, cream, broth, salt.

Ingredients:

• 2 (6.5 oz) cans of minced clams, with juice
• 2 medium potatoes, peeled and diced
• 1 cup heavy cream
• 1 cup low•sodium chicken or vegetable broth
• 1/2 teaspoon salt

Instructions:

1. In a large pot or Dutch oven, combine the canned clams (including the juice), diced potatoes, heavy cream, broth, and salt.

2. Bring the mixture to a simmer over medium heat, stirring occasionally.

3. Reduce the heat to low and let the chowder simmer for 15•20 minutes, or until the potatoes are tender.

4. Taste and adjust the seasoning with additional salt if needed.

5. Serve the clam chowder hot, garnished with extra chopped parsley if desired.

This clam chowder recipe uses just 5 main ingredients • clams, potatoes, cream, broth, and salt. The potatoes provide substance and texture, while the cream creates a rich, creamy base. The clams add protein and flavor without being too heavy. This makes for a comforting, easy•to•digest meal that is suitable for those following a diverticulitis•friendly diet.

80. Fish Soup:
White fish, broth, carrots, celery, salt.

Ingredients:

• 1 lb white fish fillets (such as cod, tilapia, or halibut), cut into 1•inch pieces
• 4 cups low•sodium chicken or vegetable broth
• 2 carrots, peeled and sliced
• 2 celery stalks, sliced
• 1/2 teaspoon salt

Instructions:

1. In a large pot, combine the broth, sliced carrots, and sliced celery. Bring the mixture to a simmer over medium heat.

2. Add the white fish pieces to the pot and continue simmering for 10•12 minutes, until the fish is cooked through and flakes easily with a fork.

3. Stir in the salt and taste, adjusting the seasoning if needed.

4. Serve the fish soup hot, garnished with extra chopped parsley or dill if desired.

This fish soup recipe uses just 5 main ingredients • white fish, broth, carrots, celery, and salt. The vegetables add fiber and nutrients, while the fish provides a lean protein source. The broth keeps the soup light and easy to digest. This makes for a nourishing, diverticulitis•friendly meal.

81. Caesar Salad: Romaine lettuce, Caesar dressing, croutons, parmesan cheese, lemon.

Ingredients:

- 1 head romaine lettuce, chopped
- 1/2 cup Caesar dressing
- 1/2 cup homemade or store•bought croutons
- 1/4 cup grated parmesan cheese
- 1 lemon, cut into wedges

Instructions:

1. In a large salad bowl, combine the chopped romaine lettuce.

2. Drizzle the Caesar dressing over the lettuce and toss gently to coat.

3. Sprinkle the grated parmesan cheese over the top of the salad.

4. Add the croutons and toss the salad again lightly.

5. Serve the Caesar salad immediately, with lemon wedges on the side for squeezing over the top.

This simplified Caesar salad recipe uses just 5 main ingredients • romaine lettuce, Caesar dressing, croutons, parmesan cheese, and lemon. The dressing, cheese, and croutons provide flavor without being too heavy, while the lemon adds a bright, acidic note. This makes for a light, easy•to•digest salad that is suitable for those following a diverticulitis•friendly diet.

82. Greek Salad: Cucumbers, tomatoes, feta cheese, olives, olive oil.

Ingredients:

- 1 cucumber, diced
- 2 tomatoes, diced
- 1/2 cup crumbled feta cheese
- 1/4 cup pitted kalamata olives, halved
- 2 tablespoons olive oil

Instructions:

1. In a large salad bowl, combine the diced cucumbers and tomatoes.

2. Sprinkle the crumbled feta cheese over the top of the vegetables.

3. Add the halved kalamata olives.

4. Drizzle the olive oil over the salad and toss gently to coat.

5. Serve the Greek salad immediately, or refrigerate until ready to serve.

This Greek salad recipe uses just 5 main ingredients • cucumbers, tomatoes, feta cheese, olives, and olive oil. The vegetables provide fiber and nutrients, while the feta and olives add flavor without being too heavy. The olive oil dressing helps bind the salad together. This makes for a light, refreshing, and easy•to•digest meal that is suitable for those following a diverticulitis•friendly diet.

83. Caprese Salad: Tomatoes, mozzarella, basil, olive oil, balsamic vinegar.

Ingredients:

• 3 tomatoes, sliced
• 8 oz fresh mozzarella cheese, sliced
• 1/4 cup fresh basil leaves
• 2 tablespoons olive oil
• 1 tablespoon balsamic vinegar

Instructions:

1. Arrange the sliced tomatoes and mozzarella cheese on a serving platter or plate.

2. Scatter the fresh basil leaves over the top of the tomatoes and cheese.

3. Drizzle the olive oil and balsamic vinegar over the salad.

4. Season with a pinch of salt and pepper, if desired.

5. Serve the Caprese salad immediately, or refrigerate until ready to serve.

This Caprese salad recipe uses just 5 main ingredients • tomatoes, mozzarella, basil, olive oil, and balsamic vinegar. The tomatoes and basil provide freshness, while the mozzarella adds creaminess. The olive oil and balsamic vinegar create a simple, yet flavorful dressing. This makes for a light, easy•to•digest salad that is suitable for those following a diverticulitis•friendly diet.

84. Cobb Salad:
Lettuce, chicken, bacon, avocado, egg.

Ingredients:

• 6 cups chopped romaine lettuce
• 1 cooked chicken breast, diced
• 2 hard•boiled eggs, sliced
• 1 avocado, diced
• 2 slices cooked bacon, crumbled

Instructions:

1. In a large salad bowl, arrange the chopped romaine lettuce.

2. Top the lettuce with the diced cooked chicken breast, sliced hard•boiled eggs, diced avocado, and crumbled cooked bacon.

3. Serve the Cobb salad as•is, or you can drizzle a light vinaigrette dressing over the top if desired.

This Cobb salad recipe uses just 5 main ingredients • lettuce, chicken, eggs, avocado, and bacon. The chicken and eggs provide protein, while the avocado adds healthy fats. The bacon provides a savory, crunchy element. This makes for a satisfying, nutrient•dense salad that is suitable for those following a diverticulitis•friendly diet.

85. Tuna Salad:
Tuna, mayonnaise, celery, salt, pepper.

Ingredients:

• 2 (5 oz) cans of tuna, drained
• 1/4 cup mayonnaise
• 1/2 cup diced celery
• 1/4 teaspoon salt
• 1/4 teaspoon ground black pepper

Instructions:

1. In a medium bowl, combine the drained tuna, mayonnaise, diced celery, salt, and black pepper.

2. Mix everything together until the tuna is well coated and the ingredients are evenly distributed.

3. Taste and adjust the seasoning as needed, adding more salt, pepper, or mayonnaise to your preference.

4. Serve the tuna salad on its own, on top of lettuce or greens, or as a sandwich filling.

This tuna salad recipe uses just 5 main ingredients • tuna, mayonnaise, celery, salt, and pepper. The mayonnaise provides creaminess, while the celery adds a nice crunch. The salt and pepper season the salad without being too heavy. This makes for a light, easy•to•digest meal that is suitable for those following a diverticulitis•friendly diet.

86. Chicken Salad:
Chicken, mayonnaise, celery, salt, pepper.

Ingredients:

• 2 cups cooked and shredded chicken
• 1/2 cup mayonnaise
• 1/2 cup diced celery
• 1/4 teaspoon salt
• 1/4 teaspoon ground black pepper

Instructions:

1. In a medium bowl, combine the shredded cooked chicken, mayonnaise, diced celery, salt, and black pepper.

2. Mix everything together until the chicken is well coated and the ingredients are evenly distributed.

3. Taste and adjust the seasoning as needed, adding more salt, pepper, or mayonnaise to your preference.

4. Serve the chicken salad on its own, on top of lettuce or greens, or as a sandwich filling.

This chicken salad recipe uses just 5 main ingredients • chicken, mayonnaise, celery, salt, and pepper. The mayonnaise provides creaminess, while the celery adds a nice crunch. The salt and pepper season the salad without being too heavy. This makes for a light, easy•to•digest meal that is suitable for those following a diverticulitis•friendly diet.

87. Egg Salad:
Eggs, mayonnaise, salt, pepper, mustard.

Ingredients:

• 6 hard•boiled eggs, chopped
• 1/4 cup mayonnaise
• 1 teaspoon Dijon mustard
• 1/4 teaspoon salt
• 1/4 teaspoon ground black pepper

Instructions:

1. In a medium bowl, combine the chopped hard•boiled eggs, mayonnaise, Dijon mustard, salt, and black pepper.

2. Mix everything together until the eggs are well coated and the ingredients are evenly distributed.

3. Taste and adjust the seasoning as needed, adding more salt, pepper, or mayonnaise to your preference.

4. Serve the egg salad on its own, on top of lettuce or greens, or as a sandwich filling.

This egg salad recipe uses just 5 main ingredients • eggs, mayonnaise, Dijon mustard, salt, and pepper. The mayonnaise provides creaminess, while the mustard adds a subtle tang. The salt and pepper season the salad without being too heavy. This makes for a light, easy•to•digest meal that is suitable for those following a diverticulitis•friendly diet.

88. Fruit Salad:
Apples, bananas, grapes, orange juice, honey.

Ingredients:

- 2 apples, diced
- 2 bananas, sliced
- 1 cup grapes, halved
- 1/4 cup orange juice
- 1 tablespoon honey

Instructions:

1. In a large bowl, combine the diced apples, sliced bananas, and halved grapes.

2. Drizzle the orange juice and honey over the fruit.

3. Gently toss the fruit salad to coat everything evenly with the orange juice and honey.

4. Serve the fruit salad immediately, or refrigerate until ready to serve.

This fruit salad recipe uses just 5 main ingredients • apples, bananas, grapes, orange juice, and honey. The orange juice and honey provide a light, sweet dressing without being too heavy. The variety of fruits offers different textures and nutrients. This makes for a refreshing, easy•to•digest dessert or snack that is suitable for those following a diverticulitis•friendly diet.

89. Potato Salad:
Potatoes, mayonnaise, mustard, salt, pepper.

Ingredients:

• 3 lbs potatoes, peeled and diced
• 1/2 cup mayonnaise
• 1 tablespoon Dijon mustard
• 1/2 teaspoon salt
• 1/4 teaspoon ground black pepper

Instructions:

1. Place the diced potatoes in a large pot and cover with water. Bring to a boil and cook until the potatoes are tender, about 15•20 minutes.

2. Drain the cooked potatoes and let them cool completely.

3. In a large bowl, combine the cooled potatoes, mayonnaise, Dijon mustard, salt, and black pepper.

4. Gently mix everything together until the potatoes are evenly coated with the dressing.

5. Taste and adjust the seasoning as needed, adding more salt, pepper, or mayonnaise to your preference.

6. Refrigerate the potato salad for at least 30 minutes before serving to allow the flavors to meld.

This potato salad recipe uses just 5 main ingredients • potatoes, mayonnaise, Dijon mustard, salt, and pepper. The mayonnaise provides creaminess, while the mustard adds a subtle tang. The salt and pepper season the salad without being too heavy. This makes for a light, easy•to•digest side dish that is suitable for those following a diverticulitis•friendly diet.

90. Pasta Salad:
Pasta, olive oil, tomatoes, mozzarella, basil.

Ingredients:

• 8 oz pasta (such as penne or fusilli), cooked and cooled
• 2 tablespoons olive oil
• 1 cup cherry tomatoes, halved
• 1 cup diced fresh mozzarella cheese
• 1/4 cup chopped fresh basil leaves

Instructions:

1. In a large bowl, combine the cooked and cooled pasta, olive oil, halved cherry tomatoes, diced mozzarella cheese, and chopped fresh basil.

2. Toss everything together gently until the pasta salad is evenly coated with the olive oil.

3. Taste and adjust the seasoning as needed. You can add a pinch of salt and pepper if desired.

4. Refrigerate the pasta salad for at least 30 minutes before serving to allow the flavors to meld.

This pasta salad recipe uses just 5 main ingredients • pasta, olive oil, tomatoes, mozzarella, and basil. The olive oil provides a light dressing, while the tomatoes, mozzarella, and basil add freshness and flavor. This makes for a refreshing, easy•to•digest pasta salad that is suitable for those following a diverticulitis•friendly diet.

91. Mashed Potatoes:
Potatoes, butter, milk, salt, pepper.

Ingredients:

• 3 lbs russet or Yukon Gold potatoes, peeled and cut into 1•inch chunks
• 4 tablespoons unsalted butter
• 1/2 cup milk
• 1 teaspoon salt
• 1/4 teaspoon ground black pepper

Instructions:

1. Place the peeled and diced potatoes in a large pot and cover with cold water.

2. Bring the pot to a boil over high heat, then reduce the heat and simmer for 15•20 minutes, until the potatoes are very tender when pierced with a fork.

3. Drain the cooked potatoes in a colander and return them to the pot.

4. Add the butter, milk, salt, and pepper to the pot. Use a potato masher or electric hand mixer to mash the potatoes until smooth and creamy.

5. Taste the mashed potatoes and adjust the seasoning as needed, adding more salt, pepper, or a splash of milk if desired.

6. Serve the mashed potatoes hot.

This mashed potato recipe uses just 5 main ingredients • potatoes, butter, milk, salt, and pepper. The butter and milk add creaminess, while the salt and pepper season the potatoes. This makes for a comforting, easy•to•digest side dish that is suitable for those following a diverticulitis•friendly diet.

92. Steamed Vegetables:
Carrots, broccoli, cauliflower, salt, olive oil.

Ingredients:

- 2 carrots, peeled and sliced
- 1 head broccoli, cut into florets
- 1 head cauliflower, cut into florets
- 1/2 teaspoon salt
- 1 tablespoon olive oil

Instructions:

1. Fill a large pot with about 1 inch of water and bring it to a boil over high heat.

2. Place the sliced carrots, broccoli florets, and cauliflower florets in a steamer basket or colander that fits inside the pot.

3. Carefully lower the steamer basket or colander into the boiling water, making sure the water doesn't touch the bottom.

4. Cover the pot and steam the vegetables for 5•7 minutes, until they are tender but still crisp.

5. Remove the steamed vegetables from the pot and transfer them to a serving bowl.

6. Drizzle the olive oil over the vegetables and sprinkle with the salt. Toss gently to coat.

7. Serve the steamed vegetables warm.

This steamed vegetable recipe uses just 5 main ingredients • carrots, broccoli, cauliflower, salt, and olive oil. The steaming method preserves the nutrients and texture of the vegetables, while the olive oil and salt provide simple seasoning. This makes for a light, easy•to•digest side dish that is suitable for those following a diverticulitis•friendly diet.

93. Garlic Bread:
White bread, garlic, butter, parsley, salt.

Ingredients:

• 8 slices white bread
• 4 cloves garlic, minced
• 4 tablespoons unsalted butter, softened
• 2 tablespoons chopped fresh parsley
• 1/4 teaspoon salt

Instructions:

1. Preheat your oven to 400°F. Line a baking sheet with foil or parchment paper.

2. In a small bowl, combine the minced garlic, softened butter, chopped parsley, and salt. Mix well until evenly incorporated.

3. Spread the garlic•butter mixture evenly over one side of each slice of bread.

4. Arrange the bread slices, butter•side up, on the prepared baking sheet.

5. Bake for 8•10 minutes, until the bread is lightly toasted and the butter is melted.

6. Serve the garlic bread warm.

This garlic bread recipe uses just 5 main ingredients • white bread, garlic, butter, parsley, and salt. The butter and garlic provide the classic flavor, while the parsley adds a fresh, herbal note. This makes for a simple, easy•to•digest side dish that is suitable for those following a diverticulitis•friendly diet.

94. Rice Pilaf:
White rice, broth, butter, onion, garlic.

Ingredients:

1. White rice
2. Chicken or vegetable broth
3. Olive oil
4. Onion
5. Garlic

Instructions:

1. In a saucepan, heat the olive oil over medium heat.

2. Add the diced onion and minced garlic. Sauté until the onion is translucent, about 5 minutes.

3. Add the white rice and stir to coat with the oil.

4. Pour in the broth and bring to a boil.

5. Reduce heat to low, cover and simmer for 15•20 minutes, or until the rice is tender and the liquid is absorbed.

6. Fluff the rice with a fork before serving.

This simplified recipe avoids ingredients that may be difficult to digest for someone with diverticulitis, such as butter. The key components are white rice, broth, olive oil, onion, and garlic • all of which are gentle on the digestive system. This rice pilaf can be a nutritious and easy•to•prepare option for those managing diverticulitis.

95. Coleslaw:
Cabbage, mayonnaise, vinegar, sugar, salt.

Ingredients:

1. Cabbage
2. Plain Greek yogurt
3. Apple cider vinegar
4. Honey
5. Salt

Instructions:

1. Shred or finely chop the cabbage and place it in a large bowl.

2. In a small bowl, whisk together the Greek yogurt, apple cider vinegar, and honey until well combined.

3. Pour the dressing over the cabbage and toss to coat evenly.

4. Season with salt to taste.

5. Cover and refrigerate for at least 30 minutes to allow the flavors to meld.

This simplified coleslaw recipe avoids ingredients that may be difficult to digest for someone with diverticulitis, such as regular mayonnaise and sugar. The key components are cabbage, Greek yogurt, apple cider vinegar, honey, and salt • all of which are gentle on the digestive system.

The Greek yogurt provides a creamy texture without the heaviness of mayonnaise, while the apple cider vinegar and honey offer a balanced tangy•sweet flavor. This coleslaw can be a refreshing and easy•to•prepare side dish for those managing diverticulitis.

96. Macaroni and Cheese:
Pasta, cheese, milk, butter, salt.

Ingredients:

1. Elbow macaroni (or other small pasta shape)
2. Shredded cheddar cheese
3. Unsweetened almond milk
4. Olive oil
5. Salt

Instructions:

1. Cook the macaroni according to the package instructions until al dente. Drain and set aside.

2. In a saucepan, combine the shredded cheddar cheese and unsweetened almond milk. Heat over medium, stirring frequently, until the cheese is melted and the mixture is smooth.

3. Add the cooked macaroni to the cheese sauce and stir to coat the pasta evenly.

4. Drizzle a small amount of olive oil over the top and gently mix to incorporate.

5. Season with salt to taste.

6. Serve hot.

This simplified macaroni and cheese recipe avoids ingredients that may be difficult to digest for someone with diverticulitis, such as regular milk and butter. The key components are pasta, cheddar cheese, unsweetened almond milk, olive oil, and salt • all of which are gentle on the digestive system.

The unsweetened almond milk provides a creamy texture without the heaviness of regular milk, while the olive oil adds a subtle richness without the potential irritation of butter. This macaroni and cheese dish can be a comforting and easy•to•prepare meal for those managing diverticulitis.

97. Roasted Potatoes:
Potatoes, olive oil, salt, pepper, rosemary.

Ingredients:

1. Potatoes, cut into 1•inch cubes
2. Olive oil
3. Salt
4. Garlic powder
5. Thyme (fresh or dried)

Instructions:

1. Preheat your oven to 400°F (200°C).

2. In a large bowl, toss the cubed potatoes with the olive oil until they are evenly coated.

3. Sprinkle the salt and garlic powder over the potatoes and toss again to distribute the seasonings.

4. Arrange the seasoned potato cubes in a single layer on a baking sheet.

5. Sprinkle the fresh or dried thyme over the potatoes.

6. Roast the potatoes for 25•30 minutes, or until they are tender and golden brown, flipping them halfway through the cooking time.

7. Serve the roasted potatoes hot.

This simplified roasted potatoes recipe avoids ingredients that may be difficult to digest for someone with diverticulitis, such as black pepper. The key components are potatoes, olive oil, salt, garlic powder, and thyme • all of which are gentle on the digestive system.

The garlic powder and thyme provide flavor without the potential irritation of fresh herbs, while the olive oil helps to create a crispy exterior on the potatoes. This roasted potatoes dish can be a nutritious and easy•to•prepare side for those managing diverticulitis.

98. Creamed Spinach:
Spinach, cream, butter, salt, pepper.

Ingredients:

1. Fresh spinach, washed and chopped
2. Unsweetened almond milk
3. Olive oil
4. Garlic powder
5. Salt

Instructions:

1. In a large skillet, heat the olive oil over medium heat.

2. Add the chopped spinach and sauté until it's wilted, about 2•3 minutes.

3. Pour in the unsweetened almond milk and stir to combine.

4. Sprinkle the garlic powder and salt over the spinach mixture, and stir to incorporate.

5. Simmer the creamed spinach for 5•7 minutes, or until the sauce has thickened slightly.

6. Serve the creamed spinach warm.

This simplified creamed spinach recipe avoids ingredients that may be difficult to digest for someone with diverticulitis, such as cream and butter. The key components are spinach, unsweetened almond milk, olive oil, garlic powder, and salt • all of which are gentle on the digestive system.

The unsweetened almond milk provides a creamy texture without the heaviness of regular cream, while the olive oil adds a subtle richness without the potential irritation of butter. The garlic powder and salt provide flavor without the potential irritation of black pepper. This creamed spinach dish can be a nutritious and easy•to•prepare side for those managing diverticulitis.

99. Glazed Carrots:
Carrots, butter, brown sugar, salt, pepper.

Ingredients:

1. Carrots, peeled and sliced
2. Olive oil
3. Honey
4. Cinnamon
5. Salt

Instructions:

1. Preheat your oven to 400°F (200°C).

2. In a large bowl, toss the sliced carrots with the olive oil until they are evenly coated.

3. Spread the carrots in a single layer on a baking sheet.

4. Drizzle the honey over the carrots and sprinkle the cinnamon and salt over the top.

5. Roast the carrots for 20•25 minutes, or until they are tender and caramelized, stirring halfway through the cooking time.

6. Serve the glazed carrots warm.

This simplified glazed carrots recipe avoids ingredients that may be difficult to digest for someone with diverticulitis, such as butter and black pepper. The key components are carrots, olive oil, honey, cinnamon, and salt • all of which are gentle on the digestive system.

The honey provides a natural sweetness to balance the carrots, while the cinnamon adds a warm, comforting flavor without the potential irritation of black pepper. The olive oil helps to create a caramelized, glazed texture on the carrots. This glazed carrots dish can be a nutritious and easy•to•prepare side for those managing diverticulitis.

100. Baked Beans: Beans, brown sugar, ketchup, mustard, bacon.

Ingredients:

1. Canned navy beans, drained and rinsed
2. Maple syrup
3. Dijon mustard
4. Onion, diced
5. Salt

Instructions:

1. Preheat your oven to 350°F (175°C).

2. In a large bowl, combine the drained and rinsed navy beans, maple syrup, Dijon mustard, and diced onion. Stir to mix well.

3. Transfer the bean mixture to a baking dish.

4. Bake the beans for 30•40 minutes, or until the sauce has thickened and the beans are heated through.

5. Remove the baked beans from the oven and season with salt to taste.

6. Serve the baked beans warm.

This simplified baked beans recipe avoids ingredients that may be difficult to digest for someone with diverticulitis, such as brown sugar, ketchup, and bacon. The key components are navy beans, maple syrup, Dijon mustard, onion, and salt • all of which are gentle on the digestive system.

The maple syrup provides a natural sweetness to balance the beans, while the Dijon mustard adds a tangy flavor without the potential irritation of regular mustard. The diced onion adds depth of flavor without the need for additional seasonings. This baked beans dish can be a nutritious and easy•to•prepare side for those managing diverticulitis.

101. Smoothie: Banana, almond milk, honey, vanilla extract.

Ingredients:

1. Banana, frozen
2. Unsweetened almond milk
3. Greek yogurt
4. Cinnamon
5. Honey

Instructions:

1. In a blender, combine the frozen banana, unsweetened almond milk, and Greek yogurt.

2. Add a sprinkle of cinnamon and a drizzle of honey.

3. Blend the ingredients until smooth and creamy.

4. Pour the smoothie into a glass and enjoy.

This simplified smoothie recipe avoids ingredients that may be difficult to digest for someone with diverticulitis, such as vanilla extract. The key components are banana, unsweetened almond milk, Greek yogurt, cinnamon, and honey • all of which are gentle on the digestive system.

The frozen banana provides natural sweetness and a creamy texture, while the unsweetened almond milk and Greek yogurt add protein and creaminess without the potential irritation of regular milk. The cinnamon adds a warm, comforting flavor, and the honey provides a touch of sweetness.

This smoothie can be a nutritious and easy•to•prepare option for those managing diverticulitis, as it's packed with fiber, protein, and other beneficial nutrients.

102. Fruit Juice: Apples, oranges, carrots, water.

Ingredients:

1. Apples, cored and chopped
2. Oranges, peeled and segmented
3. Carrots, peeled and chopped
4. Water
5. Lemon juice (optional)

Instructions:

1. In a blender or juicer, combine the chopped apples, orange segments, and chopped carrots.

2. Add water to the mixture, starting with 1/2 cup and adjusting the amount to your desired consistency.

3. If desired, add a splash of lemon juice to help balance the sweetness.

4. Blend or juice the ingredients until smooth.

5. Pour the fruit juice into glasses and serve immediately.

This simplified fruit juice recipe avoids any additional sweeteners or preservatives that may be difficult to digest for someone with diverticulitis. The key components are apples, oranges, carrots, water, and optional lemon juice • all of which are gentle on the digestive system.

The combination of apples, oranges, and carrots provides a naturally sweet and nutrient•dense juice, while the water helps to dilute the concentration of sugars. The optional lemon juice can help to balance the sweetness and provide a refreshing tartness.

This fruit juice can be a hydrating and nourishing beverage for those managing diverticulitis, as it's rich in fiber, vitamins, and minerals without any added ingredients that may cause further digestive discomfort.

103. Herbal Tea: Chamomile, honey, lemon, water.

Ingredients:

1. Chamomile tea bags
2. Honey
3. Lemon, sliced
4. Ginger, sliced (optional)
5. Water

Instructions:

1. Bring the water to a boil in a kettle or saucepan.

2. Place the chamomile tea bags in a teapot or large mug.

3. Pour the hot water over the tea bags and let them steep for 5•7 minutes.

4. Remove the tea bags and stir in a spoonful of honey to taste.

5. Add a few slices of lemon and, if desired, a few slices of fresh ginger.

6. Serve the herbal tea warm.

This simplified herbal tea recipe avoids any additional ingredients that may be difficult to digest for someone with diverticulitis. The key components are chamomile tea, honey, lemon, and water • all of which are gentle on the digestive system.

The chamomile tea provides a soothing and calming effect, while the honey adds a natural sweetness without the potential irritation of sugar. The lemon provides a refreshing tartness, and the optional ginger can help to settle the stomach.

This herbal tea can be a comforting and nourishing beverage for those managing diverticulitis, as it's hydrating and contains anti•inflammatory properties that may help to alleviate digestive discomfort.

104. Lemonade: Lemon, water, sugar, ice.

Ingredients:

1. Lemons, juiced
2. Water
3. Honey
4. Mint leaves (optional)
5. Ice

Instructions:

1. In a pitcher, combine the freshly squeezed lemon juice and water. Start with a 1:4 ratio of lemon juice to water and adjust to taste.

2. Stir in honey to sweeten the lemonade, starting with 2•3 tablespoons and adding more to your desired level of sweetness.

3. If desired, add a few fresh mint leaves to the pitcher for a refreshing, herbal flavor.

4. Fill glasses with ice and pour the lemonade over the ice.

5. Serve the lemonade chilled.

This simplified lemonade recipe avoids the use of regular sugar, which may be difficult to digest for someone with diverticulitis. The key components are lemon juice, water, honey, mint leaves (optional), and ice • all of which are gentle on the digestive system.

The honey provides a natural sweetener that is easier to digest than refined sugar. The lemon juice adds a tart and refreshing flavor, while the optional mint leaves can provide a soothing, herbal note.

This lemonade can be a hydrating and nourishing beverage for those managing diverticulitis, as it's rich in vitamin C from the lemons and contains anti•inflammatory properties from the honey and mint.

105. Ginger Tea: Ginger, honey, lemon, water.

Ingredients:

1. Fresh ginger, peeled and sliced
2. Honey
3. Lemon, sliced
4. Cinnamon (optional)
5. Water

Instructions:

1. In a saucepan, bring the water to a boil.

2. Add the sliced ginger to the boiling water and let it simmer for 5•10 minutes, allowing the ginger to infuse the water.

3. Remove the saucepan from the heat and stir in a spoonful of honey to taste.

4. Add a few slices of lemon to the tea.

5. If desired, sprinkle a pinch of cinnamon over the top.

6. Serve the ginger tea warm.

This simplified ginger tea recipe avoids any additional ingredients that may be difficult to digest for someone with diverticulitis. The key components are fresh ginger, honey, lemon, cinnamon (optional), and water • all of which are gentle on the digestive system.

The ginger provides anti•inflammatory properties and can help to soothe the digestive system, while the honey adds a natural sweetness without the potential irritation of refined sugar. The lemon provides a refreshing tartness, and the optional cinnamon can add a warm, comforting flavor.

This ginger tea can be a nourishing and soothing beverage for those managing diverticulitis, as it's hydrating and contains ingredients that may help to alleviate digestive discomfort.

106. Iced Tea: Tea bags, water, lemon, honey.

Ingredients:

1. Black tea bags or herbal tea bags
2. Water
3. Lemon, sliced
4. Honey
5. Ice

Instructions:

1. Bring the water to a boil in a saucepan or kettle.

2. Place the tea bags in a heat•proof pitcher or container.

3. Pour the boiling water over the tea bags and let them steep for 5•7 minutes.

4. Remove the tea bags and stir in a spoonful of honey to taste.

5. Add sliced lemon to the tea.

6. Fill glasses with ice and pour the iced tea over the ice.

7. Serve the iced tea chilled.

This simplified iced tea recipe avoids any additional ingredients that may be difficult to digest for someone with diverticulitis. The key components are black or herbal tea bags, water, lemon, honey, and ice • all of which are gentle on the digestive system.

The tea provides antioxidants and hydration, while the lemon adds a refreshing tartness. The honey serves as a natural sweetener, providing a soothing and anti•inflammatory effect.

This iced tea can be a refreshing and nourishing beverage for those managing diverticulitis, as it's hydrating and contains ingredients that may help to alleviate digestive discomfort.

107. Apple Cider: Apples, cinnamon, sugar, water.

Ingredients:

1. Apples, cored and sliced
2. Cinnamon sticks
3. Honey
4. Lemon juice
5. Water

Instuctions:

1. In a large pot, combine the sliced apples, cinnamon sticks, and water.

2. Bring the mixture to a boil, then reduce the heat and let it simmer for 30•45 minutes, or until the apples are very soft.

3. Remove the pot from the heat and use a potato masher or immersion blender to mash the apples, releasing their juices.

4. Strain the apple mixture through a fine•mesh sieve, pressing on the solids to extract as much liquid as possible.

5. Stir in honey to taste, starting with 2•3 tablespoons and adding more as desired.

6. Add a splash of lemon juice to balance the sweetness.

7. Serve the apple cider warm or chilled.

This simplified apple cider recipe avoids the use of regular sugar, which may be difficult to digest for someone with diverticulitis. The key components are apples, cinnamon, honey, lemon juice, and water • all of which are gentle on the digestive system.

The apples provide natural sweetness, while the cinnamon adds a warm, comforting flavor. The honey serves as a natural sweetener, and the lemon juice helps to balance the flavors.

This apple cider can be a nourishing and soothing beverage for those managing diverticulitis, as it's rich in antioxidants and contains ingredients that may help to alleviate digestive discomfort.

108. Berry Smoothie: Berries, yogurt, honey, water.

Ingredients:

1. Mixed berries (such as blueberries, raspberries, and blackberries)
2. Plain Greek yogurt
3. Unsweetened almond milk
4. Honey
5. Cinnamon (optional)

Instructions:

1. In a blender, combine the mixed berries, Greek yogurt, and unsweetened almond milk.

2. Drizzle in a spoonful of honey to taste.

3. If desired, add a sprinkle of cinnamon for extra flavor.

4. Blend the ingredients until smooth and creamy.

5. Pour the smoothie into glasses and serve immediately.

This simplified berry smoothie recipe avoids any additional ingredients that may be difficult to digest for someone with diverticulitis. The key components are berries, Greek yogurt, unsweetened almond milk, honey, and optional cinnamon • all of which are gentle on the digestive system.

The berries provide natural sweetness and antioxidants, while the Greek yogurt adds protein and creaminess without the potential irritation of regular milk. The unsweetened almond milk helps to thin out the smoothie and provide further hydration, and the honey serves as a natural sweetener.

The optional cinnamon can add a warm, comforting flavor without the potential irritation of other spices.

This berry smoothie can be a nutritious and easy•to•digest option for those managing diverticulitis, as it's packed with fiber, protein, and other beneficial nutrients.

109. Coconut Water: Coconut, water.

Ingredients:

1. Young green coconuts
2. Water
3. Lime juice (optional)
4. Ice (optional)
5. Mint leaves (optional)

Instructions:

1. Carefully open the young green coconuts and drain the coconut water into a pitcher or container.

2. If desired, add a squeeze of fresh lime juice to the coconut water for a touch of tartness.

3. Stir the coconut water to combine.

4. Serve the coconut water over ice, garnished with fresh mint leaves, if desired.

This simplified coconut water recipe avoids any additional ingredients that may be difficult to digest for someone with diverticulitis. The key components are young green coconuts, water, and the optional lime juice, ice, and mint leaves • all of which are gentle on the digestive system.

The coconut water provides natural hydration and electrolytes, while the lime juice (if used) adds a refreshing tartness. The ice and mint leaves are optional additions that can provide a cooling and refreshing element to the drink.

This coconut water can be a nourishing and hydrating beverage for those managing diverticulitis, as it's free of any added sugars or preservatives that may cause further digestive discomfort.

110. Orange Juice: Oranges, water, sugar.

Ingredients:

1. Oranges, peeled and segmented
2. Water
3. Lemon juice (optional)
4. Honey (optional)
5. Ice (optional)

Instructions:

1. In a blender, combine the peeled and segmented oranges with water. Start with a 1:1 ratio of oranges to water and adjust to your desired consistency.

2. If desired, add a splash of lemon juice to help balance the sweetness of the oranges.

3. If you prefer a sweeter juice, stir in a spoonful of honey to taste.

4. Blend the ingredients until smooth.

5. Pour the orange juice over ice, if desired, and serve immediately.

This simplified orange juice recipe avoids the use of regular sugar, which may be difficult to digest for someone with diverticulitis. The key components are oranges, water, lemon juice (optional), and honey (optional) • all of which are gentle on the digestive system.

The oranges provide natural sweetness and a rich source of vitamin C, while the water helps to dilute the concentration of sugars. The optional lemon juice can add a refreshing tartness, and the honey can provide a natural sweetener if desired.

This orange juice can be a hydrating and nourishing beverage for those managing diverticulitis, as it's rich in vitamins and minerals without any added ingredients that may cause further digestive discomfort.

111. Chicken Broth:
Chicken, water, salt, pepper, bay leaf.

Ingredients:

1. Chicken (whole or parts)
2. Water
3. Onion, diced
4. Garlic, minced
5. Salt

Instructions:

1. In a large pot, place the chicken and cover with water.

2. Add the diced onion and minced garlic to the pot.

3. Bring the mixture to a boil, then reduce the heat and let it simmer for 1•2 hours, or until the chicken is cooked through and the broth is flavorful.

4. Remove the chicken from the pot and set it aside.

5. Season the broth with salt to taste.

6. Strain the broth through a fine•mesh sieve to remove the onion and garlic.

7. Use the broth immediately or store it in the refrigerator for up to 1 week or in the freezer for up to 3 months.

This simplified chicken broth recipe avoids ingredients that may be difficult to digest for someone with diverticulitis, such as black pepper and bay leaves. The key components are chicken, water, onion, garlic, and salt • all of which are gentle on the digestive system.

The onion and garlic provide flavor without the potential irritation of additional herbs and spices. The salt helps to enhance the overall taste of the broth.

This chicken broth can be a nourishing and soothing base for soups, stews, or simply enjoyed on its own for those managing diverticulitis, as it's easy to digest and provides essential nutrients.

Thank you for joining us on this culinary journey through **_"5-Ingredient Diverticulitis-Friendly Meals: 110+ Simple Recipes"_**. We hope this book has shown you that managing diverticulitis doesn't mean sacrificing taste or spending hours in the kitchen. With just five ingredients or fewer, you can create delicious, nutritious meals that are gentle on your digestive system.

Embracing Simplicity and Health

By focusing on simplicity and health, you've taken a significant step toward better managing your diverticulitis. These recipes are designed to be easy to prepare, ensuring you can enjoy wholesome, home-cooked meals without the stress and hassle of complex cooking. We believe that good food is foundational to good health, and our goal has been to provide you with the tools to achieve both.

Continuation of Your Journey

The recipes in this book are just the beginning. We encourage you to experiment with the ingredients and techniques you've learned, adapting them to your preferences and dietary needs. Remember, the key to a successful diverticulitis diet is to listen to your body and choose foods that support your well-being.

Building a Supportive Lifestyle

Beyond the recipes, consider the broader lifestyle choices that can support your health. Regular exercise, adequate hydration, and stress management are all crucial components of living well with diverticulitis. Combine these practices with the meals from this book to create a holistic approach to your health.

Gratitude and Encouragement

We are grateful for the opportunity to support you on your path to better health. Your commitment to managing your condition and improving your diet is commendable. We hope the meals in this book bring you joy, satisfaction, and, most importantly, relief from diverticulitis symptoms.

Thank you for choosing this book and for prioritizing your health. Here's to many more meals that are simple, delicious, and supportive of your well-being.

Happy cooking!

www.ingramcontent.com/pod-product-compliance
Lightning Source LLC
Chambersburg PA
CBHW062355220526
45472CB00008B/1813